Multiple Sclerosis

Theory and Practice for Nurses

Multiple Sclerosis

Theory and Practice for Nurses

An interdisciplinary approach to providing patient-centred
care for people with MS and their families

MEGAN BURGESS, BSc, PG Dip, RGN

*MS Specialist Nurse, Greater Manchester Neuroscience Centre,
Hope Hospital, Salford*

W
WHURR PUBLISHERS
LONDON AND PHILADELPHIA

First published 2002 by
Whurr Publishers Ltd
19b Compton Terrace, London N1 2UN, England
325 Chestnut Street, Philadelphia PA19106, USA

British Library Cataloguing in Publication Data

A catalogue record for this book is available from the British Library.

ISBN 1 86156 297 7

Printed and bound in the UK by Athenaeum Press Limited, Gateshead, Tyne & Wear.

It is our choices, Harry, that show what we truly are, far more than our abilities
(Professor Dumbledore talking to Harry Potter in J.K. Rowling,
Harry Potter and the Chamber of Secrets)

For David, my Merlin and Rebecca, my sunlight –
I couldn't have done it without you.

Contents

Preface   ix

Acknowledgments   xi

Introduction   xiii

Chapter 1   1

The natural history of MS

Chapter 2   20

Diagnosing MS

Chapter 3   41

Types of MS

Chapter 4   55

Disease modifying therapies

Chapter 5   72

Symptoms and their treatments

Chapter 6   101

Bladder and bowel symptoms in MS

Chapter 7   121

Sexuality and pregnancy

Chapter 8   137

Cognitive dysfunction and depression in MS

Chapter 9   **150**

Patient-centred nursing in MS

Chapter 10   **163**

Health promotion and self-management for people with MS

Chapter 11   **184**

Complications and management of severe MS

Chapter 12   **205**

The future for people with MS

Appendix I: Resources   210
Appendix II: Glossary   217
References   224
Index   237

Preface

It is hoped this book will serve as a comprehensive resource for nurses whose working lives brings them into contact with people with multiple sclerosis (MS) and their families.

MS is no longer a disease for which nothing can be done; more and more research, treatments and therapies are being developed. All of these can be brought together to help people with MS achieve a better quality of life.

The aim of this book is to develop the reader's knowledge and skills in both the theoretical and practical aspects of caring for people with MS and to encourage the reader to apply this knowledge to their practice. The book is written with an emphasis on interdisciplinary, patient-centred nursing.

In my work both as a ward sister and as a specialist nurse, I have come to appreciate how much the needs of people with MS and their families vary and are constantly changing. This makes nursing someone with MS both challenging, and when we get it right, very rewarding. We can and do make a difference.

This book aims to provide the nurse with the knowledge they need to 'get it right' and hopefully to make a difference in meeting the challenge of MS.

Acknowledgments

Many people have helped me to write this book in many different ways; particular thanks must go to the following: Dr Cizy Mathew, Shirley Hughes, Sylvia Moss (physiotherapist) John Pauls, Dr Paul Talbot and Dr Eilis McCarthy (clinical psychologist) for their comments on various sections and encouragement of the project as a whole.

My friends and colleagues, Lorraine Lawton (Sapphire nurse) and Carol Cromwell (Parkinson's Disease Specialist Nurse) have been a source of continual support – they have made the difficult times better. Lisa Dunn (Practice Development Nurse) has been invaluable in providing advice, support and a listening ear; she has also managed to read through everything I have written and offer constructive criticism which has been gladly received.

Huge thanks must also go to my parents. My father, Roger Emlyn Roberts, has done much of the typing for me while my mother, Barbara (herself a nurse), has also read all my deliberations and has given me advice and encouragement in equal parts, despite finally moving to their long wished for country retreat. Both have been an invaluable source of support, solace, comfort and love and have shared their rural retreat willingly with a sometimes distraught daughter cum author – thank you.

My husband, David Francis and daughter, Rebecca Myfanwy, also deserve more thanks than I can convey – for their patience, forbearance, tolerance and most of all their love and support.

Last but by no means least I must say thank you to all the people with MS and their families and friends with whom I have had the privilege to work. They have taught me so much. Thank you.

Introduction

This book is written with the intention of providing nurses with a comprehensive text that can be used to inform their practice when they are caring for people with MS and their families.

MS varies so much between individuals and impacts on family members in many different ways. People with MS have many different needs and in order to meet these needs effectively, I believe it is important that we practise holistic, interdisciplinary and patient-centred care. This philosophy has shaped the way the book is written.

The extent of our understanding of aspects of MS such as epidemiology, pathophysiology and symptom management is described. This is then placed in the context of the individual with MS and the care they need from the interdisciplinary team. Patient case studies and vignettes are included where relevant. It is hoped these will aid the nurse in gaining a greater understanding of the needs of people with MS and so enable them to move closer to practising holistic, patient-centred care.

The book takes the reader through the different aspects of MS, from the historical perspective, through diagnosis and types of MS. An extensive review of the symptoms and treatments of MS follows. These chapters examine each symptom holistically in tune with the philosophy of the book. The roles of the different team members of the interdisciplinary team are also discussed in the context of each symptom. The role of the nurse specifically is emphasised throughout the book.

The book finishes with a chapter exploring the state of current research and the implications of this for the future of MS, both in terms of treatments and for nurses.

As described above case studies and vignettes are used throughout to illustrate various points and place the disease in context. Contact numbers and websites of relevant charities and other resources are included in Appendix I. There is also a glossary (Appendix II) which serves not only to explain terms used within the text but is also intended to be used as a quick reference guide.

The book is designed to be read as a whole, but, each chapter can also stand alone and can be dipped into to address a specific query.

I hope the book is useful in both informing your practice and in providing a context for some of the needs of people with MS. As nurses we are in an excellent position to provide advice, support and information in whatever way and at whatever stage of the disease people need it. This book aims to help you meet the challenge of nursing people with MS with confidence, understanding and hope.

CHAPTER 1

The natural history of multiple sclerosis

Introduction

Multiple sclerosis (MS) is the commonest cause of neurological disability in young adults. It is most commonly diagnosed between the ages of 20 and 45 years – the age many of us are settling down and beginning families and careers. It follows an uncertain and unpredictable course and prognosis for an individual diagnosed with MS varies dramatically from one person to another.

All these factors make nursing someone with MS and their family a particular challenge. The more knowledge and understanding we have of this disease, the more comprehensive and holistic will be our care. This chapter provides the background and context for the rest of the book. It does not contain practical advice on the management of people with MS but hopefully contains the answers to some of the questions we are asked in our work with people with MS and their families.

A historical perspective

Early reports of multiple sclerosis

It is unclear when MS first became extant, Robert Carswell (1838) described the first confirmed case of MS a little over 150 years ago in 1838. There are however some reports of cases prior to this, notably that of a fourteenth-century saint (Medaer, 1979). Saint Lidwina was born in 1380 in Holland and was described at the age of 12 as 'healthy and charming'. By 1396 she was only able to walk with support and three years later her walking had deteriorated further and she had developed a paresis (ie. weakness) of her right arm and was blind in her right eye. Soon

1

after this St Lidwina became unable to walk and was noted to have 'disturbances in the sensibility'. Over the next few years she enjoyed a few periods of partial relief when she reportedly experienced heavenly visions. However her illness continued to progress and she developed swallowing difficulties and died in 1433 aged 53 years of age.

Her skeleton was discovered in 1947 and studied some years later. Scientists at the time were able to prove that she had paralysis of both legs and her right arm. Medaer concluded this was proof of a central nervous system lesion with symptomatology corresponding 'strikingly to clinical criteria nowadays indicative of MS'.

Certainly St Lidwina's unfortunate history could be said to fit the symptoms of MS; however other authors have since reviewed the evidence and are not convinced (Compston, 1998c). The clinical picture alone is not sufficient to interpret her illness as MS and as the skeletal evidence verified only a central nervous system lesion we shall probably never know the truth of this particular case.

From the time of St Lidwina to the 1800s there is little or no mention anywhere of any potential cases of MS. It is unclear why this is: either MS only became recognised as a distinct syndrome at this time or the cases described by Carswell and his contemporaries were the first to appear. There are two schools of thought on this matter. It is certainly possible that there were problems distinguishing MS from other disorders of the central nervous system, e.g. tertiary syphilis, which was common in the 1800s. However as Frederikson and his colleague noted, MS was described as 'peculiar' and a 'mysterious affliction' which they felt suggested it was a new disease (Frederikson and Kam-Hansen, 1989). The early 1800s were a very active time in terms of trade, exploration and wars which would fit well with the theory that MS is caused in part by a transmissible virus. However, as is often the case with MS, things are not this simple.

Nineteenth-century pathology

To return to Robert Carswell, a renowned physician and pathologist, in 1838 he published detailed diagrams of the topography and macroscopic structure of the lesions of MS found at autopsy in the brain and spine. Almost simultaneously although working separately, Cruveillhier did the same. However Cruveillhier was able to link these lesions with the emerging clinical description of MS.

Work continued studying the pathology of affected individuals and in the 1860s Charcot took up the study of what he later named 'sclerose en plaques'. Jean-Martin Charcot is the man credited with laying the foundations for our modern knowledge of MS. Throughout his career he made many observations on the clinical presentation of MS as well as making major contributions towards the understanding of the pathophysiology. Although others before him had recognised the pathology, Charcot was the first to put a name to the disease.

Charcot was able to relate lesions observed in the spine at autopsy to particular symptoms he had observed in life. However he also noted that not all the observed symptoms could be attributed directly to lesion position, for example tremor. He proposed that this was due to the loss of conduction in part of the central nervous system and in this was well ahead of his time. He described the pathology of the lesions in some detail reporting his observations regarding loss of myelin and localised inflammation, although he did not appreciate the significance of the inflammatory response at the time.

The first personal accounts of MS

Augustus D'Este who was the illegitimate grandchild of King George III gave the first confirmed, personal account of living with MS. His illness started in 1822 and he kept a diary of his symptoms until his death in 1848 (McDonald, 1993). As with many people today, Augustus presented with bilateral optic neuritis which resolved spontaneously and then recurred four years later. 1827 was a difficult year: he experienced recurring diplopia, weakness in his legs and perineal numbness. He tells us that he was 'never able to run fast or dance' (Compston, 1998c). The following year things progressed further and Augustus developed unpleasant sensory symptoms, fatigue, urinary retention, impotency and constipation. Despite these problems he was still able to continue with his military career.

By 1843 Augustus was ataxic, numb from the waist down and suffering from nocturnal spasms. It appears that he deteriorated quite quickly from this point as he became paralysed and lost the use of both arms before dying in 1848. The account he left of his life with MS describes many of the problems faced by people today and is notable only by being the first such account.

He also leaves an account of the various medications he was prescribed which included silver, mercury, arsenic, opium and antimony.

These were all standard medications of the time. Accounts of MS by physicians or patients were rare in the early 1800s and merited single case reports being published in the medical journals of the day; Charcot himself observed and reported only 37 cases throughout his career, not many at all by today's standards. However by the end of the nineteenth century MS had become one of the most common causes of admission to a neurological ward, as it is today. It is still not entirely clear whether this represents an increasing incidence or whether, as is more likely, this apparent explosion of cases represents an increasing recognition and understanding of the signs and symptoms of MS (Compston, 1998c).

Developments during the late nineteenth and early twentieth centuries

During the late nineteenth and early twentieth centuries work to understand better the pathophysiology of MS carried on apace. In 1863 Rindfleisch observed that each plaque contained a blood vessel at its centre (Rindfleisch, 1863, cited in Compston, 1998c) he rightly concluded that the blood vessels were synonymous with local, chronic inflammation at the site.

Over the next 40 years or more, work on understanding the structure of the central nervous system in general continued. Neuroglia were recognised as the supporting structures for nerve cells (literally 'nerve glue') and were noted to play a role in tissue repair. Oligodendrocytes were recognised as a distinct sub-group of cells (Robertson, 1899) and in 1913 it became evident that they were responsible for making myelin within the central nervous system (Cajal, 1913). All this ensured a solid foundation on which to build.

In 1933 Russell Brain, a highly respected neurologist, published the first edition of *Diseases of the Nervous System*, later editions of which still form a valued reference for neurologists today. By following Brain's descriptions of MS through successive editions of his work it is possible to chart the development of our understanding of MS over time (Compston, 1998c). In the first edition he describes the sequence of plaque formation; he notes the phagocytosis of myelin with subsequent overgrowth of fibrous glial cells and axonal loss. Brain also observed what he described as 'shadow plaques' although he did not understand their significance. (It is now known that these represent areas of partial, spontaneous remyelination.) With respect to the natural history of the disease, Brain reported statistics describing incidence and prevalence and commented on the uneven geographic and racial distribution of the disease.

A fairly complete description of the clinical picture is included and he concludes by suggesting that an understanding of immunity would lead to a cure for MS. Today it is well recognised that MS is an immune mediated disease and much research in this area is ongoing.

Origins of the MS Society

By 1945 the general public was becoming more aware of MS. On 1 May 1945 an advert appeared in the personal column of the *New York Times* asking anyone with MS to get in touch. The number of responses was huge and the Association for the Advancement of Research into MS was set up and this soon evolved into the MS Society. The UK MS Society was founded in 1952 with two main aims, i.e. to promote and fund research in MS and to provide welfare and support for individuals with MS and their families. These aims hold good today and the MS Society remains an essential source of information and support as well as being responsible for funding many different projects. Most recently it has become involved in political lobbying for equal access to treatment and services for people with MS throughout the United Kingdom.

Douglas McAlpine was present at the formation of the MS Society and in 1955 produced a book entitled *Multiple Sclerosis* (McAlpine *et al.*, 1955). It is only since then that consistency of nomenclature has been achieved. This has become a classic textbook on MS and the authors have not lost sight of the impact of MS and are able to relate their work to the lives and experiences of patients and their families.

The last 50 years

Over the last 50 years there has been a rapid growth in our understanding of MS although this remains incomplete. In the 1960s it was demonstrated that partial remyelination of the axons in the central nervous system does occur. Further work has confirmed this and shown that although remyelination occurs it is only partial and the myelin is inappropriately thin (Prineas *et al.*, 1993). This leads to a partial recovery of conduction along the axons and accounts for the recovery often observed following a relapse.

Other studies (McDonald, 1993) of affected axons found that transmission of impulses was prolonged so that messages along the nerves were not relayed accurately. It was also reported that extended activity of the affected axons could result in temporary conduction block, i.e. an effective shutting down of the nerve, reversible after rest. These findings readily explain the myriad of different symptoms which people with MS experience.

The 1980s saw further breakthroughs. In 1981 magnetic resonance imaging (MRI) was shown to be extremely sensitive in detecting lesions in MS (Young *et al.*, 1981). Brains from patients at post-mortem were scanned and showed that the gross pathology of the lesions corresponded to the abnormalities detected on the scans. The use of MRI as a tool both for research and to aid diagnosis has been vital. While a positive MRI scan is not definitive of MS, looked at in conjunction with other tests and clinical findings it can greatly increase the neurologist's confidence in a diagnosis of MS. This has in turn meant that people now receive a confirmed diagnosis much sooner than was previously possible.

The 1990s have seen further development of our understanding of MS. The profile of MS among health care professionals, researchers and the general public is greater than ever and services for people with MS are continuing to grow and develop.

Interferons and their impact on provision of care for people with MS

In December 1995 Betaferon was licensed in the UK having been licensed two years previously in America (R&D Focus, 1994). Two other interferon betas, Avonex and Rebif followed. Interferon betas are the first medications that actually affect the course of the disease. All three have been shown to reduce the number of relapses experienced by an ambulatory individual with relapsing-remitting MS. Betaferon is also licensed for use with people who have secondary progressive disease and it has been shown that it can slow down progression of the disease (European Study Group, 1998). While the interferon betas represent a major breakthrough, they are not without controversy and their use will be discussed at length in Chapter 4.

Indirectly interferon beta has also been instrumental in raising the standard of services for people with MS and their families generally. Patients prescribed interferon need training in self-injection technique and ongoing support and monitoring while on treatment. This created a need for MS specialist nurses and their numbers have grown from single figures in the mid 1990s to over 80 at present and are continuing to rise. MS specialist nurses cover all aspects of care, including education and research. MS nurses also serve as a specialist resource for other health care professionals.

In 1997 the MS Society published a set of standards of care (Freeman *et al.*, 1997) which was developed after extensive consultation with health care professionals and people with MS and their families. This document sets out the minimum standards of care people should expect at different stages in the disease process. This is the first document of its kind and underlines increasing recognition of the importance of the interdisciplinary team in caring for people with MS.

Historically prognosis for people with MS was gloomy and it was widely felt that nothing could be done to help. However, with our ever increasing understanding of MS in terms of cause, pathology, natural history, treatment and interdisciplinary input we now know this is far from true. As McDonald stated in his Charcot Lecture 'the time has now come, not to prevent but to have reasonable prospects of curtailing and ameliorating the effects of the disease' (McDonald, 1993). It is hoped that the next 20–30 years will see us move beyond curtailing and ameliorating into a time when we can prevent and cure MS.

Epidemiology of MS

Why study epidemiology?

Epidemiology is the study of the natural history of a disease, i.e. the how, where and when of disease occurrence. The sort of data that may be collected includes patient characteristics, presenting symptoms, socio-economic status of patients and distribution in time and place of the disease (Wade, 1996).

Fox stated that 'the basic premise of epidemiology is that the disease does not occur randomly but in patterns which reflect the operation of the underlying causes' (Fox, 1970). Thus, by understanding the reasons MS is distributed in a particular pattern, we should be able to determine the cause of MS and so be much closer to controlling the disease. Epidemiological studies also allow us to have a fuller appreciation of prognosis for people diagnosed with MS and can help us to better understand the different types of MS and the pathogenesis of disease onset (Rudge, 1999).

The questions asked by epidemiologists are also just the sort that patients and their families ask and while the field is complex with no definitive answers, it is worth gaining a basic knowledge of the subject so we can inform our patients accordingly.

There are few diseases whose epidemiology has been studied as extensively as MS. Unfortunately, despite the extensive research so far undertaken, the answers to many of the questions are still not clear. We do know that MS is a chronic, demyelinating disease, which may lead to considerable disability in some people, and that the underlying pathology is caused largely by an immune response.

Before looking in more detail at some of the relevant studies, it is important to be aware that there are problems inherent in any epidemiological study of MS. One of the first difficulties is in defining the population to be studied. Initially databases of patients of individual neurologists were used but these were neither inclusive nor random (Rudge, 1999). It is necessary therefore to define the population geographically and endeavour to trace every individual with MS in that area. This is unlikely to be straightforward, as not everyone with MS will be within the health care system. Records from many different sources should be reviewed including private clinics and MS Society records if possible. No matter how exhaustively records are tracked down, the end result depends on the quality of the existing records and of the diagnosis.

This leads us to the second confounding factor in this type of study. The number of people diagnosed with MS in any given area depends upon the availability of a neurologist and the criteria used in making a diagnosis, both of which tend to vary in time and place. This may give rise to an apparent increase in incidence that should more accurately be attributed to an increase in recognition. For example, a comprehensive study in Iceland found evidence of a significant increase in incidence of MS. At the time this was interpreted as being indicative of an epidemic and therefore of an infectious causative agent (Kurtzke et al., 1982). However it later became apparent that the increase in incidence also coincided with the arrival of the first neurologist to be based in Iceland which is now felt to be the most likely explanation for the sudden increase in incidence.

The third problem to be considered when designing an epidemiological survey of people with MS is also connected with diagnosis. Due to the nature of the disease and the potential difficulties in obtaining a confirmed diagnosis, there is usually a time lag between onset of symptoms and diagnosis. This tends to average 3–5 years where there is good health care provision (Riise, 1997). Therefore, any survey of people with MS in a given area will not detect those with most recent onset of disease and the figures can only be taken as accurate for the time period 3–5 years prior to the end of the survey.

Before looking at some of the conclusions researchers have been able to draw from studies to date, some terminology is needed. There are three basic measures used in epidemiology:

Incidence: Number people developing MS in 1 year in a defined area

Prevalence: Number people with MS in a defined area at a given time

Frequency: Incidence
                    ───
           Number people at risk in same population in 1 year/per 100,000

Note the difference between incidence and prevalence, incidence being the number of new cases in any one year and prevalence being the total number of people with MS in a defined area at a particular time. Note that frequency also depends on the number of people in the total population who are at risk which in MS is age-dependent (20–59 years). The proportion of the population fitting this age range will vary over time as the age distribution of the population alters and this may be a further confounding factor.

While frequency gives us the best estimate of risk in a given population, it must always be borne in mind that incidence data is only reliable several years later due to the problems with time lag. Therefore, most studies use prevalence data, as this is slightly easier to obtain. However it is not a good measure of risk, figures given will always be lower than actual figures and will be affected by time lag; by survival rates locally and by migration in and out of the population. This makes it difficult to compare prevalence rates in different populations, which in part accounts for some of the anomalies found in many studies of distribution of MS around the world (Sadovnick and Ebers, 1993).

How is MS distributed?

There are few diseases in the world, which have such a wealth of information available about prevalence and incidence worldwide. The distribution is non-random and appears to follow certain patterns which over the years have led to many different theories as to the cause of MS. As yet the full picture remains incomplete but advances in our understanding have been made and the jigsaw is slowly being pieced together.

As a general rule of thumb, the prevalence of MS becomes higher with increasing distance from the equator. While MS tends to be rare in countries such as Africa and equatorial America, it is relatively common in northern

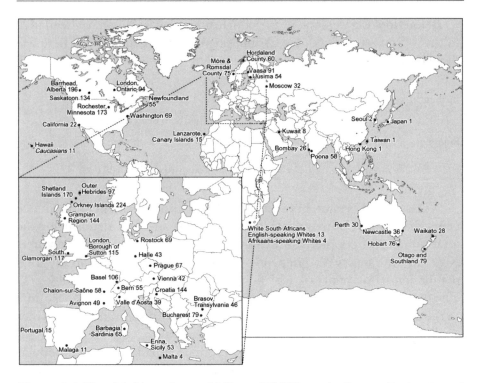

Figure 1.1 The global prevalence of MS per 100,000 people. Source: Environmental Factors in Multiple Sclerosis. Proceedings of the MS forum Modern Management Workshop, Montreal, Canada. October 1998, Worthing: PPS Europe, 1999.

Europe, northern America and southern Australia (see Figure 1.1). On closer inspection it has become evident that the areas of high prevalence tend to be those with large populations of northern European origin (Ebers *et al.*, 1998). It has been proposed that this pattern of distribution is possibly due to settlement of these areas by the Vikings. Subsequent migration of the descendants of these populations could explain the observed distribution i.e. sizeable migrations from northern Europe to both Australia and America (Poser, 1995). However, the patterns are too complex, with too many anomalies for this to represent more than a small part of the whole picture.

The prevalence around the world varies dramatically from less than 5/100,000 to more than 150/100,000 people. Figures can vary significantly over very short distances e.g. Sicily (53.3/100,000) and Malta (4/100,000) (see Figure 1.1).

In the UK there are approximately 85,000 people with MS. Prevalence varies from 115/100,000 in Surrey to 170/100,000 in the Shetlands. The Orkneys have a particularly high prevalence rate at 224/100,000 population (Ebers *et al.*, 1998). It is unclear at present why the Orkneys should have such a high prevalence; they are, however, a well-defined and much studied population. Recent surveys have shown some levelling off of the south to north gradient as methodology becomes standardised and diagnostic criteria refined. It remains likely, however, that there is a genuine gradient effect with north-east Scotland continuing to have a higher prevalence, albeit somewhat less pronounced than previously thought (Compston, 1998a).

Studies have also shown that the ratio of males to females with MS remains constant at 1:2 as does age of onset. Age of onset of MS tends to be a year or two later in men than in women but men are more likely to develop severe disease. The average age of onset is 29–33 years although people may be diagnosed at almost any age. It is likely that people diagnosed in later life (e.g. two gentlemen in my own caseload both recently diagnosed with MS in their 70s) have had a mild form of the disease for many years and it is only as symptoms become more troublesome that people seek help. Conversely an increasing number of children are being diagnosed with MS although this remains rare with less than 0.3% people having onset of symptoms before the age of 10 (Sadovnick and Ebers, 1993).

What do the studies tell us?

Due to the inherent patterns in the distribution of MS around the world, many researchers have proposed an environmental factor as a possible causative agent. One of the earliest authors to propose infection as being responsible was Pierre-Marie in 1884 (Marie, 1884). Indeed many authors since have produced evidence in support of this (e.g. Kurtzke and Hyllested, 1988). However the likelihood of a single infectious agent being implicated is slim; not least because no organism has been isolated which fits the necessary criteria.

As our understanding of genetics grew, the search for a cause shifted from environmental agents to population genetics. This work continues today although it is now thought likely that our genetic make-up accounts for only one-third of the risk of developing MS. It is probable that the remaining two-thirds of risk is made up of exposure to an environmental factor(s). The element of chance should not be overlooked either, the coincidence of a particular series of risk factors combining to produce a susceptible individual is likely to play a part (Ebers *et al.*, 1998).

Below is a summary of the most influential studies to date and a review of the way they have shaped our understanding.

Twin studies

Studies of twins, one or both of whom have MS, are of particular interest to researchers. In theory, if genes are solely responsible for determining our risk of developing MS then if one monozygotic twin is diagnosed with MS there should be a 100% chance that the other twin will also develop MS. However the actual risk in this instance has been shown to be around 25% (Sadovnick *et al.*, 1993). This indicates that genetic factors only account for less than one-third of the total risk.

It is important to stress at this point that MS is not hereditary. This is something patients are understandably anxious about, particularly when first diagnosed. As already noted, genes do play a part in MS and while occasional family clusters occur, it is much more common to observe individuals developing MS with no previous family history of the disease. Table 1.1 gives a rough approximation of risk of developing MS for relatives of individuals diagnosed with MS. Work in this area is ongoing.

Table 1.1 Age-adjusted risk of developing MS for relatives of an individual already diagnosed

Relative	Age-adjusted risk (%)
Parent	2.0
Sibling	3.8
Child	1.8
Nephew/niece	1.6
Aunt/uncle	0.9
First cousin	0.9

Source: Robertson *et al.* (1996).

Migration studies

The other main focus of epidemiological studies relevant to genetics is migration. Again there is a rule of thumb that can be used; an individual migrating as an adult carries their original risk of developing MS with them. If they migrate as a child, they acquire a risk closer to that of their new home. A UK study looked at children of West Indians who had emigrated to parts of London and the West Midlands. It showed that while the parents retained the low risk of developing MS as found in the West Indies, children who moved before the age of 15 developed a higher risk of being diagnosed with MS more in line with that found locally (Dean and Elian, 1997).

Environmental factors

Thus it became evident that while studying the genetics of people with MS is important, other factors must be implicated and researchers have turned again to examine possible environmental factors. The present emphasis is to look for a combination of both genetic and environmental factors, which may play a part in the onset of MS.

Some of the different environmental components studied include: climate, diet, geology, local industry, sanitation, pollutants and of course infection. Of these some have proved more likely than others; none, however, has shown the same degree of linkage as exists between prevalence and latitude (Ebers *et al.*, 1998). Those factors showing most consistent associations are climate and diet.

Several studies show that a combination of cold temperatures and/or humidity can be correlated with an increasing prevalence of MS (Norman *et al.*, 1983). It is unclear why this should occur although there is some evidence linking lack of vitamin D3. Vitamin D3 is synthesised in the skin by ultra-violet light from sunlight and is also found in fish. It has been proposed that vitamin D3 is required for the biosynthesis of myelin in the central nervous system and that it also acts as a regulator of inflammatory immune responses (Goldberg, 1974). This is no more than a hypothesis at present but circumstantial evidence is compelling. Vitamin D3 levels have been inversely correlated with increasing severity of MS (Nieves *et al.*, 1994).

This ties in with studies looking at diet. An increased consumption of smoked and cured meats and less convincingly, animal fats have been linked with increased risk (Lauer, 1997). It should be stressed that it is too early to draw conclusions from these studies and that research into this area is ongoing.

The evidence for an infectious agent remains inconclusive but is a continuing notion. To date no infectious agents have been isolated consistently from MS tissues. This does not necessarily mean that an infective agent is not implicated; it may be that the infection is present but not yet recognised; or that it is not present in the central nervous system but elsewhere in the body or there may be several different agents responsible.

Summary

The epidemiology of MS is a fascinating and complex field. By understanding the epidemiology of MS it is hoped that we will understand the causes of the disease itself. Studying people with MS in any particular region is not without its pitfalls and these should be borne in mind when reviewing any research.

The prevalence of MS is strongly correlated with latitude, increasing with distance from the equator. It has been shown that the risk of an individual developing MS is multi-factorial. While the disease is not hereditary, there is a genetic component thought to make up approximately 25% of an individual's risk factor. The remaining risk is probably due to one or more environmental triggers and probably a degree of chance as well. Which environmental factors are implicated remains unclear but may include diet and climate. The role of infection as a trigger also remains unclear but cannot be ruled out.

The continued study of both genetic and environmental factors is essential. An understanding of the predisposing genetic factors will help us to unravel the immunology and pathology of the disease. An understanding of the environmental factors will assist us in minimising the risk for susceptible individuals.

Pathology of MS

In order to understand the complex processes occurring in MS, it is necessary to review normal anatomy and immunology.

Anatomy of the central nervous system

MS affects the central nervous system, i.e. the brain and spinal cord. There are a number of different cells specific to the central nervous system and these can be split into two types – neurones and glial cells. Neurones are responsible for transmitting information while glial cells form the supporting network for the neurones. The functions of each are reviewed in more detail below.

There are three types of glial cells:

1. Astrocytes: these are highly branched cells found throughout the central nervous system, they support the neurones and are an integral part of the blood–brain barrier. Astrocytes also secrete nutrients essential for some neurones and can repair damage to tissue within the central nervous system forming scars (this process is also known as gliosis) (Hutchins *et al.*, 1997).
2. Oligodendrocytes: these cells are very important in our study of MS as they are responsible for myelinating the axons. The myelin acts as

electrochemical insulation around the axon in much the same way as the plastic coating around an electric wire provides insulation when an electric current is passed through it. A single oligodendrocyte may provide myelin for up to 50 separate axons.

3. Microglia: when the cells of the central nervous system suffer any sort of injury, the microglia migrate to the site where they multiply and phagocytise (i.e. absorb) any debris.

Neurones receive, process and send information to other neurones or effector tissues elsewhere in the body. To do this they change the biochemical properties of the cell wall along their length resulting in the transmission of electrical impulses. This process is facilitated by myelin.

Neurones are composed of three basic parts, a cell body with dendrites and an axon stemming from it. The flow of information enters the neurone via the dendrites and passes through the cell body and down the axon to the synapses where it connects to the next neurone. The axons may extend a significant distance before ending in a synapse (e.g. more than 1 metre). Myelin forms in a series of segments along the length of the axon, the gap between each segment is known as the node of Ranvier (see Figure 1.2). The thickness of the myelin and the frequency of the nodes of Ranvier determine the speed of transmission along the nerve. Thus axons with a thick myelin sheath will have a much higher conduction velocity

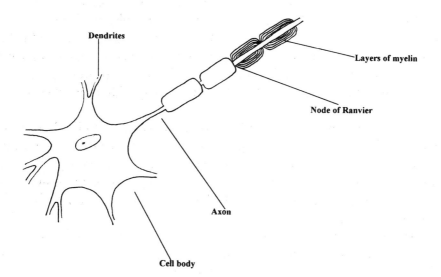

Figure 1.2 Diagram of a myelinated axon.

than ones with only a thin sheath. The transmission of electrical impulses along the neurones imposes a requirement for vast amounts of energy. The nervous system uses more oxygen and glucose than any other system in the body.

Blood–brain barrier

The blood–brain barrier is unique to the central nervous system. Blood vessels within the central nervous system differ in both structure and function from those elsewhere in the body. The endothelial cells of the blood vessel form tight junctions with high electrical resistance. They are surrounded by the foot like processes of astrocytes which form a very effective barrier against unwanted molecules or cells passing from the blood stream to the central nervous system. The barrier is further strengthened by the presence of macrophages that remain close to the cell wall of the blood vessel and have a phagocytic function. The blood–brain barrier is vital to normal functioning of the central nervous system, ensuring a highly selective transport system between the blood and the brain and spinal cord; its main function is one of protection.

Overview of the immune system

MS is known to be an immune mediated disease and in order to understand plaque formation it is necessary to understand something of the immune system. An overview of the cells of particular relevance follows.

Lymphocytes are found in lymph tissue and blood. There are two types of lymphocytes – T cells and B cells, each of which can be further subdivided. T lymphocytes (derived from the thymus gland) lie inactive in the lymph tissue until activated by an antigen (e.g. an infective agent). There are different types of T cells each having a different function (see Table 1.2).

B lymphocytes are derived from bone marrow and circulate in the blood and lymph system. When they encounter a specific antigen, they are activated and secretions from T helper cells cause them to reproduce. They go on to form either memory B cells (with the same function as memory T cells) or plasma cells which produce antibodies specific to the presenting antigen.

Antibodies are protein molecules known as immunoglobulins. By binding with an antigen, an antibody ensures it is recognised and destroyed by killer T cells and macrophages.

Table 1.2 Type and function of T lymphocytes implicated in the pathogenesis of MS

T Lymphocyte	Function
Killer T cells	Destroy antigen bearing cells
Helper T cells	Stimulate replication of B lymphocytes
	Activate other T cells
	Facilitate transformation of monocytes to macrophages
Suppresser T cells	Inhibit T helper cells
	Suppress B lymphocyte activity
Memory T cells	Retain a memory of targeted antigen so that a rapid immune response can be initiated should antigen represent

Cytokines are proteins that carry messages between cells and are secreted by T helper cells. Macrophages also secrete cytokines that promote phagocytosis. There are several different categories of which we will note only those relevant to MS, i.e. interferons.

T cells secrete interferons. There are three types of interferon, alpha, beta and gamma. Gamma interferon is produced in response to myelin antigens. A study treating patients systemically with gamma interferon found it caused a dramatic deterioration of the MS and was stopped early (Panitch *et al.*, 1987). It is thought gamma interferon attracts T cells to plaque sites (Panitch and Beuer, 1993). Alpha and beta interferons suppress the action of gamma interferon and decrease cytokine release from T cells prohibiting their replication (Arnason, 1993).

Plaque formation in MS

There are two different pathogenic processes occurring in MS that have the potential to produce neurological deficits. The first is an inflammatory process associated with demyelination. This may be accompanied by loss of axons. The mechanism is not fully understood but is thought to be related to lack of trophic support. Both processes are believed to start at the time of disease onset, however there is some limited, spontaneous remyelination at some sites which protects many of the axons initially. Any axonal loss occurring in the early stages tends not to produce neurological deficits, as the central nervous system is able to compensate. It is only when the amount of axon loss exceeds a defined threshold that permanent deficits can occur. It is thought this may account for the change from relapsing-remitting disease to secondary progressive disease (Trapp *et al.*, 1999).

Activated T cells pass through the blood–brain barrier and into the central nervous system. The activated T cells then recognise their specific antigen on nearby macrophages and microglia and secrete cytokines causing further inflammation in the locality of the blood vessel. The cytokines, including gamma interferon, break down the blood–brain barrier locally and there is further escalation of the inflammatory process.

Secretion of cytokines also causes proliferation of B-lymphocytes with antibodies specific to myelin. These antibodies are able to cross the leaky blood–brain barrier and bind to the surface of the myelin so attracting macrophages and killer T cells, which then begin to phagocytise the myelin. Cytokines and activated glial cells also help to break down the myelin further.

After an indefinite period of time, this process tends to resolve spontaneously. The reason for this is unclear although it is likely that some mechanism of T cell inhibition is involved (Hohlfeld, 1999). The type and amount of inflammation in the central nervous system varies depending on the stage of the disease process. Once the acute inflammatory process has resolved, some healing occurs and scar tissue develops. This process is known as gliosis.

These areas of gliosis, or scarring, are known as plaques. The destruction of myelin and oligodendrocytes leaves areas of naked axons. It is in these areas that transmission of messages along the axons becomes delayed or completely blocked (known as conduction block). The symptoms caused by a particular plaque depend in part on the area in which the plaque has formed. Not all plaques result in functional deficit, those that do not are known as silent plaques.

Once the local inflammatory process has settled there is some patchy remyelination by the oligodendrocytes in the surrounding area. The new myelin is much thinner than normal, however it is sufficient to provide some protection for the axons and to allow some recovery of conduction. It is uncertain what determines whether or not plaques will remyelinate although the more oligodendrocytes left intact, the more likely is remyelination (Prineas et al., 1993). Remyelination is more common during the early phases of MS (possibly because oligodendrocytes are left largely unharmed at this stage). However over time the amount of remyelination is reduced. In later stages of MS, demyelination is accompanied by widespread loss of oligodendrocytes, which leaves the axons vulnerable to toxic molecules within the local inflammatory environment, which in conjunction with lack of trophic support from neuroglia, may result in degeneration and loss of the axon (Trapp et al., 1999). This accounts for long-term neurological deficits in people with MS.

Summary

An individual who is susceptible to developing MS because of their genetic make-up is exposed to one or more unknown environmental triggers. This activates T cells outside the central nervous system allowing them to cross the blood–brain barrier. They then bind to their specific antigen within the central nervous system and secrete cytokines. The cytokines are toxic and also serve to attract more T cells and macrophages to the area. The inflammatory process causes further damage to the blood–brain barrier allowing the passage of B-lymphocytes into the central nervous system. The B-lymphocytes multiply and produce antibodies, which cause further damage to both myelin and oligodendrocytes.

Thus there is an area of inflammation surrounding a central vein with a leaky blood–brain barrier, axons are stripped of their myelin and the myelin debris is phagocytosed. The axons stripped of their insulating layer are no longer able to conduct impulses efficiently, if at all, so the potential myriad of symptoms evident in MS can result.

Remission often occurs although it is unclear what initiates this. Inflammation subsides and the blood–brain barrier repairs itself. The axons often remyelinate although repeated healing and inflammation in the same site can lead to permanent scarring and plaque formation (e.g. gliosis) (Lassmann, 1998).

CHAPTER 2

Diagnosing multiple sclerosis

Introduction

Diagnosis in multiple sclerosis is notoriously difficult. In order to make a diagnosis the neurologist must rule out any other conditions that can mimic symptoms of MS; they must also find evidence of plaques which have formed within the central nervous system separated by both time and location (Paty and Hartung, 1999).

Despite recent advances such as the use of magnetic resonance imaging (MRI), the diagnosis is still based largely on the patient's history and neurological examination. Once having reached a diagnosis of MS the neurologist is then in the difficult position of having to communicate this to the patient and their family, clearly and empathetically.

Primary care – the first point of call

While the neurologist tends to have responsibility for making the diagnosis, it is the general practitioner (GP) who is the first to see the patient. MS can present in many different ways depending on the site of plaque formation, symptoms can vary in severity and may be transitory in nature. Indeed symptoms may be so vague initially that patients themselves put their problems down to stress or perhaps a trapped nerve; as a result many people delay visiting their GP until the symptoms become troublesome or more persistent. Once patients present at their GP's surgery, they represent a major challenge. Statistically GPs would only expect to see a new case of MS every 15 years or every 100,000 patient contacts. Some GPs will go through their whole career without diagnosing a case of MS (Keen, 2000).

Most GPs have only limited experience of MS. People with MS make up approximately 1 per 1000 of the population and as most GPs have a caseload of 2000–3000 patients they are therefore likely to have only 2–3 people with MS under their care at any given time. Everyone with MS experiences the disease differently and it is therefore difficult for the GP to build up expertise in this area.

GPs do, however, have an invaluable role to play in supporting the patient and their family and particularly in recognising when someone needs referral to a specialist and in dealing with the day-to-day problems that can occur. The first and arguably most important aspect of their role is in referring patients appropriately to a neurologist so that a diagnosis can be made, thus opening the door to appropriate support and treatment for the patient and their family.

Patients can present with a wide variety of different symptoms (see Table 2.1). The majority of these symptoms are usually indicative of a diagnosis other than MS and it is vital that GPs recognise the few individuals who present with some combination of these symptoms, which warrant referral to a neurologist.

Once the GP has decided to refer an individual for further investigations it is important that the referral is made as soon as possible. In making the referral the GP should consider which hospitals locally would best meet the needs of the patient. The hospital needs to be capable of performing the appropriate diagnostic tests and of providing the necessary levels of support and follow-up post diagnosis. Ideally an MS specialist nurse should be based at the Centre (Barnes *et al.*, 1999).

Table 2.1 Common presenting symptoms in MS

- Double vision
- Blurred vision
- Poor balance and co-ordination
- Muscle weakness (often in legs)
- Stiffness or spasticity in muscles
- Altered sensation, e.g. numbness, tingling or a burning feeling
- Slurred speech
- Fatigue inappropriate to activity
- Bladder and bowel problems
- Impotence
- Forgetfulness and poor concentration

Secondary or tertiary care – the diagnostic process

Once referral to a consultant neurologist is made, the individual should be seen as soon as possible. The Standards of Health care for people with MS (Freeman *et al.*, 1997) recommend that the ideal period between referral and being seen by a neurologist should be four weeks. It is also recommended that ideally diagnostic investigations should be completed within a month of the initial appointment. Unfortunately this is not always possible and waiting times vary around the country.

The theory of the diagnostic tests and the implications for both nurse and patient are described below. The criteria used in making a diagnosis and the support that should be provided for the patient are explored later in the chapter.

Patient history

The diagnosis of MS remains primarily a clinical one; the patient history and examination are central.

When taking a history the doctor will ask about the onset and progression of the patient's symptoms; they will also ask about any relevant family history and the patient's lifestyle. They should also ascertain if the patient has experienced any other neurological symptoms in the past, the patient might need prompting with this. Often people may have experienced an episode of double vision or numbness many years ago that only gains significance in hindsight. This can be vital in establishing a definite diagnosis, as the doctor needs to be able to find evidence of two or more lesions separated in time as well as within the central nervous system. A thorough history also helps to rule out other possible diagnoses.

The nurse may be needed during the history taking to support the patient if they are distressed. On some occasions it may also be appropriate for the nurse to accompany the doctor so that she can complete her own assessment of the patient without asking the same questions over again.

Neurological examination

This normally follows on from the initial history taking. The nurse may be needed to support the patient and provide simple explanations of the various components of the examination. The nurse should also ensure that she is aware of any findings as this may have implications for the provision of care for that patient.

The different components of a neurological examination with particular relevance to MS are detailed below.

General observation

This is vital and should be ongoing. Throughout the time the doctor spends with the patient, they should be observing behaviour, general appearance, mood, cognitive processes, speech patterns, motor function etc. This can give invaluable information and clues as to the problems the patient is experiencing.

Cognitive function

This sometimes requires more formal testing and various tests are used. Orientation of the patient in time and place is important to establish. In MS, the short-term memory may be a particular problem. This can be assessed by asking the patient questions about their activities over the preceding few days or by giving the patient some names or a sequence of numbers at the beginning of the examination and asking them to recall these at the end. A thorough examination of cognitive function may not be necessary at this stage.

Cerebral function

Cerebral function is concerned with communication and recognition of objects and people. In MS, recognition is unlikely to be a problem, however, communication may be affected. It is important to distinguish between dysphasia (either receptive or expressive) and dysarthria, which is an abnormality of motor function rather than cerebral function. Cerebral function should be assessed throughout the examination.

Cranial nerves

I Olfactory nerve – test the patient's ability to detect a variety of different smells using a smell kit. This is unlikely to be affected in MS.

II Optic nerve – the patient's visual acuity should be assessed as should the extent of their visual field. Visual problems are often one of the presenting symptoms in MS. Patients may experience visual field defects, blurred or double vision or abnormalities of their colour vision. This should all be elicited through formal testing and history taking.

Ophthalmoscopic examination should also be performed. A pale optic disc indicates optic atrophy, which results from past episodes of optic neuritis.

Nerves III oculomotor, IV trochlear and VI abducens – all these nerves are tested together as they supply the muscles that control movement of the eyeball. Nystagmus may be observed in someone with MS. The patient is asked to follow the doctor's pen or finger with his gaze and when the eyeball reaches its extreme of movement (either vertically or horizontally) it may appear to flicker and jump if nystagmus is evident.

V Trigeminal nerve – this is the nerve which supplies the side of the face and both the sensory and motor components of its function should be tested. Brushing a piece of cotton wool along the side of the face can be used to test the sensory function. The trigeminal nerve also controls chewing and this can be assessed during the examination and history taking.

VII Facial nerve – this nerve controls the taste mechanisms and ensures motor control of the facial muscles. If there is a lesion affecting the muscles, asymmetry of the face will be evident.

VIII Acoustic nerve – this controls hearing and also balance (vestibular control). Hearing is very rarely affected in MS but balance maybe and will be discussed in more detail below.

IX Glossopharyngeal and X vagus nerves – together these control the gag reflex, swallowing and the vocal cords. The doctor will use a tongue depressor and ask the patient to say 'ah' while observing the uvula and soft palate, the gag reflex can also be checked by lightly touching the back of the soft palate with the tongue depressor. The voice quality and any motor problems evident when forming words (i.e. dysarthria) may indicate lesion(s) in this area.

XI Spinal accessory nerve – this nerve controls the function of the neck muscle (sternocleidomastoid muscle) and the back muscles (trapezius muscle). If a lesion is present these muscles will be weak and the doctor should test their strength by asking the patient to shrug their shoulders and move their chin against resistance. They are unlikely to be affected in MS.

XII Hypoglossal nerve – the hypoglossal nerve controls the movement of the tongue. Any fibrillations or weakness (e.g. asymmetry) of the tongue can mean a lesion affecting this nerve. This is unlikely in MS.

NB The cranial nerves themselves are classed as peripheral nerves and as such will not become demyelinated, however their site of entry within the central nervous system may be compromised.

Motor function

The patient will be asked to walk a short distance while the doctor observes their gait; the nurse should assist the patient if they are unable to manage alone. Problems that may be particularly associated with MS include footdrop, ataxia and spasticity. Footdrop occurs when the individual is unable to fully dorsi-flex the foot when walking, this can lead to the patient lifting that leg higher in order to compensate, they may also be prone to 'falling over their own feet'.

Ataxia is said to occur when an individual walks with a wide-based gait that is uncoordinated. The lay person may often mistake them as being drunk. Ataxia may occur if a cerebellar or brainstem lesion is evident.

Evaluation of muscle strength

The doctor must observe the size, tone and symmetry of the patient's muscles. Spasticity may become evident during the examination; i.e. an increased resistance to passive movement followed by a sudden easing of resistance. The patient is asked to move each limb in different directions against the doctor's hand. In someone with MS some degree of weakness is common, spasticity may be evident but is less likely in the early stages of the disease.

Sensory function

These tests examine the patient's ability to perceive different sensations with their eyes closed. The doctor touches the skin in different areas (e.g. forearm, leg, and face) with a wisp of cotton wool and with a pinprick; the patient is asked to say when and what they can feel. This may highlight areas of abnormal sensation, which are common in MS.

Proprioception is the sense by which someone determines the position of their limbs etc. relative to the rest of their body and the surrounding environment. This can be tested by asking the patient to close their eyes while the doctor moves the big toe up or down; the patient then has to tell the doctor in which direction he is moving the toe. This ability to determine position sense may be impaired in MS.

Another aspect of sensory function that can be affected in MS is the ability to recognise simple objects placed in the hand with the eyes shut (e.g. coins). This may be simply tested during the neurological examination.

Cerebellar function

The cerebellum is responsible for balance and co-ordination. There are a number of tests that the doctor can use in this context. The patient can be asked to touch the doctor's finger and their own nose in quick succession. Lower limbs can be tested by asking the patient to lie on the bed and rub the heel of one leg up and down the shin of their other leg. In both these instances the doctor will be looking for signs of tremor, ataxia and poorly co-ordinated movements, all of which may be evident in MS.

Romberg's Test also examines balance; patients are asked to stand erect and then close their eyes, if they lose their balance when they close their eyes this is said to be a positive result and implies damage to the dorsal column.

Assessment of reflexes

Each reflex is co-ordinated via a different pathway and any abnormalities detected in the reflexes can give important information regarding problems within the central nervous system.

Triceps – patient is asked to bend their arm and hold the other arm with their hand facing their body, the doctor taps the elbow with the tendon hammer and the elbow should extend. Abnormality indicates a lesion at C7-8.

Biceps – the patient should assume the same position as above, but the doctor places his fingers on the inside of the bent arm and taps these with the tendon hammer, the elbow should flex. Abnormality indicates a lesion at C5-6.

Abdominal – each side of the umbilicus, above and below, is stroked with the end of the tendon hammer. The umbilicus should move in the direction the skin is stimulated. Abnormality indicates a lesion at T8-12.

Quadriceps (knee jerk) – the doctor supports the patient's legs with an arm below their knee and the patellar tendon is struck, the knee joint should extend. Abnormality indicates a lesion at L3-4.

Babinski reflex – a moderately sharp object (e.g. a key) is stroked along the lateral aspect of the sole from the heel round to the ball of the foot. The toes will normally flex downwards (i.e. down-going plantars). If the toes extend upward (i.e. up-going plantars) then abnormality of the pyramidal tract is indicated (adapted from Hickey, 1997, pp. 103–29).

Magnetic resonance imaging (MRI)

While the diagnosis of MS remains primarily clinical, the use of magnetic resonance imaging (MRI) has had a big impact since it was first applied to MS in 1981 (Young *et al.*, 1981). As MRI has become more routine over the last few years, neurologists have been able to use it to confirm a suspected diagnosis of MS much sooner than they were able to in the past. While a MR scan is not a definitive test for MS; looked at in conjunction with the clinical picture it can provide evidence of plaques, which are clinically silent. In practice this means that neurologists are now able to confirm a diagnosis of MS much sooner than they could previously (McDonald, 1998).

MR scanners are large and make a loud knocking sound during the scan; patients have to lie very still and can find the process distressing, particularly if they suffer from claustrophobia. The radiographer and patient are able to talk to each other throughout the scan, which can help ease any anxieties. It is important that the nurse takes time to explain the procedure to the patient before they are taken to the scan room. Patient information leaflets describing the process should be made available. The MR scan is in effect a large magnet and patients will be advised to remove any metal items from their person, watches and credit cards must also be removed as they can be affected by the magnetic field. If patients have a pacemaker or other metal in their body (e.g. metal clips or heart valves) they cannot be scanned. However dental work such as fillings or metal braces do not present a problem and patients can be scanned without difficulty.

Once the patient is inside the scanner a radio wave is transmitted in short bursts at a pre-determined frequency. The radio wave causes the different tissues in the body to emit a signal that is then used to construct a black and white image of the area being scanned. Different tissues emit different signals; for example water (e.g. cerebrospinal fluid) appears white while fatty tissues (e.g. brain) appear darker. Diseased tissues often have a higher water content than the surrounding tissues and so appear lighter in colour on the scan. This is the case with plaques in MS which appear white (see Figure 2.1).

Patients may also be scanned using a contrast medium, the most common one is Gadolinium-DTPA which is well tolerated. The reason for using a contrast agent is that any breaches in the blood–brain barrier can be highlighted thus indicating an area of active MS. By scanning a patient

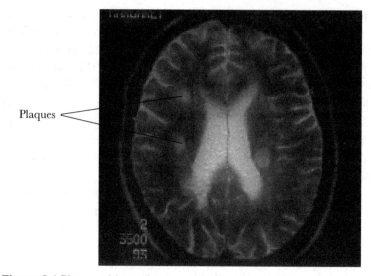

Plaques

Figure 2.1 Plaques of demyelination as seen on a magnetic resonance scan. (Supplied by Dr Jon Sussman, Greater Manchester Centre for Clinical Neurosciences).

using a contrast agent, not only is any disruption of the blood–brain barrier evident but there is also a higher number of lesions detected, which can assist in making a differential diagnosis (Schild, 1990).

It should be noted that the number of plaques seen on a MR scan does not correlate with an individual's function. Someone may have many plaques showing on their scan but the vast majority are 'silent', i.e. not clinically evident and so that the individual has few if any impairments. Alternatively an individual may have only a few plaques evident on their scan but because of the position of the plaques the individual has significant disability. It is not yet possible to predict with any accuracy the functional impairment of an individual purely by looking at the scan.

Lumbar puncture

A lumbar puncture may not always be necessary; the MR scan result together with the patient history and examination may be sufficient to make a diagnosis. However additional confirmation may well be needed and the cerebrospinal fluid analysis can provide valuable information.

A lumbar puncture is often painful and distressing for the patient and the nurse should remain with the patient throughout the procedure. During a lumbar puncture a hollow lumbar needle is inserted into the subarachnoid space between lumbar vertebra 3–4 or 4–5. It is vital that strict aseptic technique is followed throughout.

A lumbar puncture should not be performed if there is any concern that the patient may have raised intracranial pressure (this does not occur in MS) or if there is any indication of infection at the site of the lumbar puncture.

Before starting, the procedure should be explained to the patient and any questions they have should be answered fully. It is helpful if the patient empties their bladder before starting as this aids their comfort and minimises any disturbance. The patient is then asked to lie on their side on the edge of the bed. They should bring their knees up to their chest with their chin touching their knees; the nurse may need to help the patient into position.

The site is cleaned and covered with sterile drapes. A local anaesthetic (e.g. Lignocaine) should be injected. Once the needle is inserted into the subarachnoid space the stylet is removed and cerebrospinal fluid samples can be collected. A few drops are usually placed in four sterile containers labelled 1–4 with number 1 being the first sample collected and number 4 the last. This allows an assessment of the colour gradation through the samples to be made and allows differentiation between a traumatic tap and a haemorrhage to be made. A traumatic tap is said to occur when the tissues at the puncture site bleed. The first cerebrospinal fluid sample in this instance would be heavily bloodstained with each successive sample being less so. If a patient has had a subarachnoid haemorrhage the samples will be uniformly bloodstained.

Once the procedure is completed the lumbar puncture needle is removed and a sterile dressing applied to the puncture site. The patient should be made comfortable and the bed changed if necessary. The care of the individual following a lumbar puncture remains a matter for individual doctors to determine, however the consensus of opinion is that the patient must lie flat for between 6 and 24 hours afterwards (Hickey, 1997, p. 89). The patient must also be encouraged to drink 2–3 litres of clear fluids during the first 24 hours (Lisa Dunn, member of UK Benchmarking group, personal communication); an appropriate analgesia should be prescribed and administered as required. Patients may experience headaches that may be severe or mild in nature and are aggravated by sitting upright; if this occurs, the patient should be advised to lie flat and continue to drink good amounts of fluids.

During the 24 hours after the procedure, the patient's blood pressure, pulse, temperature and respirations should be recorded regularly, the puncture wound should also be checked regularly for signs of oozing. In this way potential complications of infection and cerebrospinal fluid leakage can be detected early.

Once a cerebrospinal fluid sample is obtained it is subject to a number of tests:

Culture and cell count

As a matter of routine, each cerebrospinal fluid sample will be cultured and a count of any cells present made. Cerebrospinal fluid should be clear and colourless in appearance, any organisms present may indicate an infective process and the doctor should be informed immediately. Contamination of the samples is possible and the microbiologist will advise accordingly.

Cell counts can give an indication of various disease processes:

- < 5 white blood cells per mm cubed is normal;
- 5–35 white blood cells per mm cubed can be indicative of MS;
- > 35 white blood cells per mm cubed are rare in MS and indicative of an infective process.

During a relapse in MS the number of white blood cells in the cerebrospinal fluid is often elevated, the number tends to be higher than normal during remission due to silent plaque activity.

Protein and glucose levels

These levels are normal in approximately two-thirds of people with MS but may be slightly elevated in some.

- Normal range for protein in cerebrospinal fluid: 15 – 45mg/100ml
- Normal range for glucose in cerebrospinal fluid: 60 – 80mg/100ml

Immunoglobulin G index

Immunoglobulins are naturally present in the body and are more commonly known as antibodies. Immunoglobulin G (Ig G) is the most predominant class of antibody and is produced by the immune system (i.e. B cells, see Chapter 1) when it is exposed to a specific antigen on more than one occasion. In MS the immunoglobulin crosses the blood–brain barrier and binds to the surface of the myelin, so facilitating demyelination.

Thus by measuring the amount of Ig G present in the cerebrospinal fluid, important information regarding the integrity of the blood–brain barrier can be obtained. A venous blood sample is also required to allow a comparison of Ig G in the cerebrospinal fluid with Ig G in the plasma, this comparison gives a figure called the Ig G index; 70% of people with clinically definite MS have an Ig G index of at least 0.7 (Bates *et al.*, 1993).

Oligoclonal bands

Electrophoretic testing of the cerebrospinal fluid and plasma from the venous blood sample is carried out. If Ig G has breached the blood–brain barrier and entered the cerebrospinal fluid then oligoclonal bands will be present on electrophoresis (similar to chromatography in principle). In 95% of people with MS oligoclonal bands will be present in the cerebrospinal fluid sample but not in the plasma. There is a low incidence of false positives and 5% of people with MS will be negative. However the presence of oligoclonal bands is highly indicative of MS although not definitive (Andersson *et al.*, 1994).

Evoked potentials

It is well known that demyelination slows down conduction along the axons and evoked potentials (EPs) were first applied to the study of optic neuritis in 1973 (Halliday *et al.*, 1973). Evoked potentials can be particularly useful if MRI is inconclusive as they can demonstrate the presence of otherwise silent lesions.

Visual evoked potentials (VEPs) are most commonly used. The patient is sat in front of a black and white chequer board screen and watches the flashing squares while an electroencephalograph (EEG) recording is made. The time for the flashing image to travel along the optic nerve and provoke a response recorded via the EEG is measured.

The majority of people with MS will demonstrate some delay in response. This is not specific to MS but does indicate demyelination within the optic nerve.

Auditory evoked potentials may also be performed but in practice they are less sensitive and tend to be rarely used (McDonald, 1998).

Making a diagnosis

Making a diagnosis of MS is dependent on evidence of two or more lesions being found within the central nervous system separate in time and space. The evidence used to illustrate the existence of these lesions comes from the different diagnostic tests described above. Until recently, the criteria used to make a diagnosis were known as the Poser criteria (Poser *et al.*, 1983). These described various levels of certainty of a diagnosis of MS depending on the available evidence. For example, in order to make a diagnosis of 'clinically definite MS' the individual must have had at least two relapses separated by at least a month, with evidence of two or more lesions on examination, or one lesion on examination and one from paraclinical evidence such as MRI or evoked potentials.

Other levels of certainty included 'laboratory supported definite MS'; 'clinically probable MS' and 'laboratory supported probable MS'.

When these criteria were published in 1983, our depth of understanding of MRI scans and their use as a diagnostic tool was very much in its infancy. It was only two years earlier that the first paper describing the application of MRI to MS was published (Young *et al.*, 1981). It was therefore by necessity that the Poser criteria were somewhat complex to ensure consistent use of the available diagnostic tests and to provide some standardisation of diagnosis.

However it has recently been felt necessary to reassess the existing diagnostic criteria. To this end a panel of neurologists from around the world convened with the intention of defining a diagnostic scheme that would be easy to use in clinical practice, suitable for use in clinical trials, and which would integrate MRI as an instrument uniquely sensitive to pathological changes. The panel has produced diagnostic criteria, which now supersede the Poser criteria, and these were published in July 2001 (McDonald *et al.*, 2001).

These new diagnostic criteria are relatively much simpler with only three possible outcomes from a diagnostic evaluation i.e. 'MS'; 'possible MS' (where the diagnosis is equivocal) or 'not MS'.

The basic tenets of the Poser criteria still hold, however the scheme has now been simplified somewhat due to the increased significance of MRI data. In order to make a confirmed diagnosis of MS, the individual must have had two or more attacks with objective clinical evidence of two or more lesions. In this context an attack is defined as a neurological disturbance of the kind seen in MS which lasts at least 24 hours and which is confirmed by expert clinical assessment (McDonald *et al.*, 2001).

If the individual has only had one clinically confirmed attack, the neurologist will require evidence of dissemination of plaques in time and space from either MRI alone or, if this is not evident from MRI in conjunction with the presence of oligoclonal bands and raised Ig G index in the CSF. It may sometimes be necessary to await a further clinical attack, which implicates a different site, before confirming diagnosis.

Some people will present with insidious neurological progression which is suggestive of MS, in these circumstances a positive CSF is necessary alongside evidence of dissemination in time and space from MRI, or delayed visual evoked potentials or continued progression for a year. This group of people would be diagnosed with primary progressive MS (see Chapter 3).

If these criteria cannot be met or a better explanation for the individual's signs and symptoms exists, then the diagnosis of 'not MS' should be made. There will still be some people who do not quite fit the diagnostic criteria and in this case a diagnosis of 'possible MS' should be made (McDonald *et al.*, 2001). In this circumstance it is important that a neurologist follows up the individual until an accurate diagnosis can be made or until it is evident their symptoms have resolved and are unlikely to return.

Giving a diagnosis

Having completed the diagnostic tests and reviewed the results the neurologist must then inform the patient of the diagnosis. It is recommended that the results be given to the patient within 2–4 weeks of their completion (Freeman *et al.*, 1997).

It is important that the diagnosis is explained tactfully and with an appreciation of each person's particular needs; adequate support and follow-up in the period following diagnosis must also be ensured. The way a diagnosis is given can have a huge impact on the patient and their family and can affect their coping skills for many years to come. Studies have shown that patients prefer their diagnosis to be given earlier rather than later (Robinson, 1991; Fieschi, 1999).

It should be noted that since MRI scanning has become much more readily available the majority of people with MS can be diagnosed earlier than would otherwise be possible. It is also important to realise that in the past there was no early intervention available for people with MS (e.g. interferons – see Chapter 4) and the importance of the interdisciplinary team in advising and supporting the patient and their family post-diagnosis was not fully recognised.

Most people do not suspect that they have MS prior to their diagnosis whereas the vast majority of clinicians think that they do. Thus the shock of diagnosis may be greater than the clinician anticipates and this should be borne in mind (Fieschi, 1999).

Case study 1 – How not to give a diagnosis

A young university student presented with a twelve-month history of weakness and altered sensation down her left side. She remembered an episode of double vision some two years before. She was admitted to the neurology ward and had a MR scan, a lumbar puncture and visual evoked potentials. The neurologist had some results back by the end of the week, which were enough to confirm the suspected diagnosis of MS. However, preferring to wait until all the results were back, he advised commencement of intravenous steroids over the weekend and arranged to discuss the results with the student the following week. Unfortunately the junior doctor on setting up the steroids informed the student that this was 'for her MS', the doctor then left the bedside without discussing anything further. The nurses then had to spend considerable time with the student and her family trying to calm and reassure them as best they could. The neurologist and MS specialist nurse were able to see the family on the following Monday and needed to spend considerable time with them at this stage. The student and her family have been left with a mistrust of the medical profession and a heightened anxiety regarding the MS.

Studies have shown that patients are not given enough information when informed of their diagnosis (Ford and Johnson, 1995). If patients can be given a definitive diagnosis backed up with appropriate information given at the time they have an increased sense of well being and a slightly higher quality of life than patients who are not given a definite diagnosis (Mushlin *et al.*, 1994).

Guidelines for giving a diagnosis

Various guidelines have been published to assist clinicians in telling people that they have MS (Compston *et al.*, 1993, Freeman *et al.*, 1997). These are expanded upon below.

1. Once the diagnostic tests have been completed the doctor should arrange with the patient an agreed time when the results will be explained to them; they should be given the opportunity of having a friend or relative with them at this time if they wish.
2. At the agreed time the patient with their relative or friend should be taken to a quiet room off the ward or if in a clinic setting ensure that there will be no interruptions. A nurse or therapist that the patient knows should accompany them.

3. The neurologist should give a clear and simple explanation of their test results and diagnosis. Time should be allowed for the patient and their relative to ask questions and express their anxiety.
4. It is useful if the patient's symptoms are explained in context with the MS and if a working prognosis can be given. Information should be given carefully and slowly as the patient's ability to absorb information at the time of diagnosis is very limited.
5. Written information should be given, including contact numbers for the MS Society or other local organisations. The patient should also be given a contact number for someone within the interdisciplinary team; ideally this should be the MS specialist nurse/therapist.
6. A follow-up appointment with the neurologist within 2–4 months of diagnosis should be made to allow the patient to discuss any concerns they may have.

Once the neurologist has answered all their questions as best he can, he should leave the patient and their friend/relative alone with the nurse. The nurse should then give them the opportunity to ask any further questions, people may feel more able to express their fears to the nurse than the doctor. The nurse should then give the patient the option of time alone with their relative.

During the remainder of their stay in hospital (if diagnosed as an inpatient) the patient and their family must be given the opportunity to ask questions and express their fears and concerns. If possible they should have the chance to talk to the MS specialist nurse before discharge.

On discharge patients must have a follow-up appointment with the consultant and a contact number for the MS specialist nurse or other member of the interdisciplinary team. The patient should also understand any medication that they may have been given and be informed of any referrals made to other health care professionals in the community or outpatient settings. It is helpful to provide the patient with an information sheet at discharge detailing all this information, a copy should be sent to the GP and MS specialist nurse and one kept in the notes (see example Figure 2.2).

Psychological impact of diagnosis

People react in many different ways to a diagnosis of MS but common themes emerge. Many people are shocked and anxious, some may respond with relief, most experience a mixture of positive and negative

```
Name......................          Hospital No ...................
Address .....................       Date of Birth...................
................................
Consultant.....................     Secretary......................
Telephone......................
Follow up Appointment...........
MS Specialist nurse.............    Contact number..............
Appointment.....................
MS Society Details.................................................
Welfare Rights/Citizens Advice Bureau..........................


Referrals Made
Team member(s)...................      .........................
Contact No.(s).....................    .........................
Appointment/waiting time............   .........................
Medication..................................................................
Other Information...........................................................
```

Figure 2.2 Example of an information sheet to be used on discharge for people diagnosed with MS.

emotions (Robinson, 1991). An individual's initial reaction depends to a large extent on their history and background. The period leading up to a diagnosis of MS can be fraught with uncertainty, symptoms are often vague and transitory during the early stages and patients may begin to feel (or are told) it is 'all in their mind'. Others with perhaps more intrusive symptoms may become convinced their problems are life threatening and in this context the diagnosis of MS can be a relief.

People's understanding of MS at diagnosis will also differ and the nurse should take care to ask the patient what MS means to them. Many people have very little knowledge of MS or just assume that everyone with MS quickly becomes wheelchair bound. Others may have family or friends who already have MS which will colour their own perceptions of the disease. Patients may well need reassuring that MS is not terminal or infectious and that many people with MS remain active and independent for many years after the diagnosis (Lechtenberg, 1995). Patients should also be made aware that advances have and are being made, there is now much more available in terms of treatment, therapy and support than even a few years ago.

Grieving

Despite reassurances and support it is normal for people with MS and their families to grieve for their loss of health. Many studies have been done examining the grieving process for people diagnosed with a chronic illness (Westbrook and Viney, 1982; Murray, 1995; Antonak and Livneh, 1995) and little consensus regarding the grieving process has been reached. It is likely that people each work through the grieving process in their own way and at their own speed with common themes recurring. These common themes may be experienced in any order and more than once with varying peaks of intensity (see Table 2.2). However people cope with their diagnosis, they are likely to require ongoing support from health care professionals for an extended period (Koopman and Schweitzer, 1999).

Table 2.2 Common themes experienced by people diagnosed with MS

- Shock
- Anxiety
- Denial
- Depression
- Anger
- Acknowledgement
- Adjustment

It is important that people understand that the feelings they are experiencing are normal and even necessary. Alexander Burnfield (1982), a psychiatrist with MS, writes

> Not only did I have a right but it was necessary for me to be frightened, angry, confused and sad about my predicament ... Once I discovered that it was OK ... I began to accept MS as part of me.

Ongoing support and continuity of care is vital and every member of the interdisciplinary team has a role to play. It is important to remain positive as far as possible, MS can be life-affirming as well as devastating (see Case study 2).

Case study 2 – MS can be positive

A 35-year-old mother presented with rapid onset of left-sided weakness. She is married with two daughters, 10 years and 11 years old and worked part-time as a secretary, which she hated. Her weakness quickly became so severe that she was unable to walk and not knowing what was wrong, she and her husband presented at Casualty feeling very anxious.

She was admitted to the neurology ward and underwent routine diagnostic tests. The results confirmed a diagnosis of MS; she was told of the diagnosis and commenced on steroid treatment. Her initial reaction was to request as much information as possible about MS and she was seen by the MS specialist nurse.

Over the next few weeks she had a lot of input from the interdisciplinary team, both in hospital and in the community and her weakness largely resolved. She is left with symptoms of mild left-sided weakness and fatigue; as a result she has had to leave her secretarial job.

She continued to learn as much as she could about MS. She has also taken the opportunity to spend more time with her children and to train as a counsellor, something she had always wanted to do. As well as working as a volunteer counsellor, she has also set up a support group for young people with MS in her locality. She continues to do well despite occasional setbacks.

Role of the interdisciplinary team following diagnosis

An interdisciplinary approach is important for people with MS at every stage of their life. The interdisciplinary team should provide a comprehensive and co-ordinated approach to care on an individual basis. Unfortunately the availability of services across the UK varies although standards are improving as purchasers and providers become more aware of the importance of the interdisciplinary team to all their neurology patients. Below is a brief overview of the interdisciplinary team relevant to the person newly diagnosed with MS.

Role of the GP

The GP may not be expert with regard to all aspects of MS; however, he does have a major role to play. It is vital that the GP is supportive and empathetic to the patient and their family. GPs are often very experienced at dealing with specific symptoms that may occur and should liaise with the neurologist and MS specialist nurse as needed. It is also important that GPs recognise that an individual may develop problems unconnected to MS, which will need treating in the usual way.

Role of the neurologist

The neurologist is key in diagnosing, treating and prescribing appropriate treatment for the person with MS. They should liaise with other members of the interdisciplinary team as needed and should keep the GP informed of any changes to the patient's care.

Role of the MS specialist nurse

The MS specialist nurse provides continuity of care and a point of contact for the patient and their family. They liaise closely with other members of the interdisciplinary team and make referrals to the team as necessary, they are able to bridge the gap between hospital and community. The MS nurse also has an important role to play in terms of education, both for people with MS and their families and for other health and social care professionals. Many nurses run educational courses for people newly diagnosed with MS and their partners (Brechin *et al.*, 2001) in conjunction with other members of the interdisciplinary team. The MS Society also run similar courses through many of their branches.

Role of the occupational therapist

The occupational therapist (OT) is invaluable in teaching patients how to manage fatigue both at home and in the workplace. They also assess an individual's ability to perform the activities of daily living and can provide advice, aids and adaptations which enable the individual to be as independent and active as possible.

Role of the physiotherapist

The physiotherapist offers advice and treatment on movement disorders with a view to improving mobility and maximising normal movement, therefore minimising the development of secondary musculoskeletal problems. The physiotherapist is responsible for providing walking aids and splints should these be necessary.

Role of the social worker

The social worker is key in advising people about benefits, work-related issues, housing and in providing a community care package if required. Many social workers are also trained counsellors and can play an important part in helping people with MS and their families begin to accept the changes MS has caused in their lives.

Role of the counsellor

Counsellors may be based in the hospital, GP's surgery or in the voluntary sector. Some individuals with MS and some family members will have particular difficulties in coping with the impact of MS on their lives and counselling can be invaluable in helping people to work through their fears and concerns. Newly diagnosed patients should be made aware that this service is available if required.

Support groups

MS Society of Great Britain and Northern Ireland

The MS Society is a national organisation providing information and support for people with MS, families, friends and carers. They produce a wide range of information booklets and run a help line. Local branches may have a variety of services on offer from social evenings to yoga sessions; some also run education courses for people newly diagnosed with MS entitled 'Getting to Grips'.

The MS Society is also responsible for a number of initiatives to improve the services for people with MS including the publication of the 'Standards of Healthcare for people with MS' (Freeman *et al.*, 1997).

Multiple Sclerosis Research (Charitable) Trust

The Multiple Sclerosis Research (Charitable) Trust (MSRCT) produce a range of information specifically for people newly diagnosed with MS. They are also heavily committed to providing education for nurses and other professionals with an interest in MS at whatever level it is needed. In conjunction with the Royal College of Nursing they have set up the MS Nurse Forum and provide a library and information service for interested professionals.

They are also committed to improving services for people with MS and in conjunction with the MS Society have published the *Basics of Best Practice in the Management of Multiple Sclerosis* (Barnes *et al.*, 1999).

Contact details for these and other MS related charities can be found in Appendix I.

CHAPTER 3

Types of MS

Introduction

MS varies dramatically in terms of severity and every individual follows a different and largely unpredictable course.

Some individuals have such mild disease that they never develop symptoms during their life, but are diagnosed at post-mortem having died of an unrelated condition (Herndon and Rudick, 1983). Others will have such severe disease that they develop profound disability within a couple of years of onset. It is these wide varieties of clinical course that make living with MS so difficult and caring for people with MS so challenging.

Within the many individual variations of MS, some patterns have emerged and five different types of MS have been defined. The definitions are based on the pattern of disease course an individual is likely to follow. Theoretically the advantages of defining disease type in this way are as follows:

1. The individual and their family may gain some idea of the likely course of their disease.
2. The interdisciplinary team can advise the patient and their family more appropriately with respect to treatments, aids and adaptations etc. that may be needed. The interdisciplinary team can anticipate problems and, at least in theory, plan ahead somewhat.
3. Some treatments (e.g. interferon beta and glatiramer acetate) are only helpful for people with certain types of MS.
4. Clinical trials tend to recruit patients according to their type of MS.

However, in reality, it is rarely immediately evident exactly what type of MS an individual has. It often takes two or more years before this becomes apparent and can be stated with any confidence. It should also be stressed that within each type of MS there is a wide variation in prognosis and the functional difficulties individuals are likely to experience. Treatment and support tends to be provided depending on an individual's immediate needs with some provision for the future and is rarely, if ever, provided based purely on the type of MS someone has.

Historically the terms used to describe the different types of MS were many and consensus definitions were only established in 1996 (Lublin and Reingold). These terms are explained below; it should be noted that the different types of MS tend to be described with respect to the pattern of relapses experienced although there is no consensus definition of a relapse. A reasonable working definition can be taken as a relapse being the appearance of a new symptom or the reappearance of old symptoms, which last more than 24 hours (Lublin and Reingold, 1996).

Relapsing-remitting MS

This is possibly the most widely recognised type of MS and the majority of people experience this pattern initially. An individual with relapsing-remitting disease will experience periods of acute worsening of function to varying degrees (i.e. relapse) with variable periods of recovery (i.e. remission) in between. People rarely make a 100% recovery following relapse and are often left with some residual problems, e.g. parasthesia (pins and needles) or fatigue. The periods of recovery or remission may last anything from weeks to years (see Figure 3.1).

The uncertainty and unpredictability so evident in MS is particularly so for people with relapsing-remitting disease. People may experience long periods of remission or have successive relapses within a relatively short space of time. An individual's recovery following relapse may be full or partial and there is always the fear that this time they may not recover at all. This can present particular problems in coming to terms with MS. Psychologically people can find it very difficult to cope with; they may be just beginning to accept particular functional limitations and achieve some quality of life when another relapse occurs and they are faced with a new set of problems to adjust to.

A significant proportion of people with relapsing-remitting MS go on to develop secondary progressive disease at a later stage. There appears to be little agreement between authors as to the numbers of people experiencing any particular type of MS at any given time. However it is likely that up to 85% of people with MS follow a relapsing-remitting course

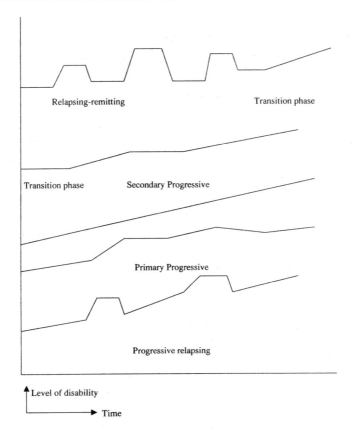

Figure 3.1 Graph to illustrate the different types of MS. After Lublin and Reingold 1996.

initially with approximately 50% of them going on to develop secondary progressive disease within 10 years (Frederikson *et al.*, 1996).

Transition phase

The transition phase is not a type of MS but is the period during which an individual who has been having well-defined relapses separated by periods of remission enters the secondary progressive phase. It can take several months or a couple of years before it is possible to state with confidence that the individual no longer has relapsing-remitting disease but is now in the secondary progressive stage.

During the transition from relapsing-remitting disease to secondary progressive MS, many people experience a difficult time both emotionally and physically. Many people will feel heightened anxiety, loss of control and fear of the future. People often tend to go through a further grieving process feeling anger, sorrow and despair. Some also feel guilty because they think they are 'letting people down' (Kalb, 2000). People in this stage, and their families, will often need a great deal of support.

Secondary progressive MS

This is said to occur when an individual who has followed an initial relapsing-remitting course switches to a more progressive course. The transition from one type to the other tends to be gradual and it is often only over time that the change becomes apparent.

The rate of progression of disability varies enormously. For some people it is very gradual while others may experience a marked progression experiencing severe functional limitations relatively quickly. At any one time approximately 60% of people with MS have secondary progressive disease (Conference Report, 1999). The loss of the improved quality of life previously experienced during remissions can be profound.

Primary progressive MS

People with primary progressive MS experience a continuous worsening of their condition from onset. This is often a gradual process but may follow a more rapid course. As well as experiencing varying rates of deterioration, some people may experience plateaux or relapses superimposed on a progressive course (see Figure 3.1).

This type of MS is much less common and only approximately 10% of people with MS have primary progressive disease (Conference Report, 1999). Due to the unremitting decline usually experienced with primary progressive MS it can be one of the most difficult types of MS to deal with for all concerned. (Further discussion of the psychological and physical problems experienced in moderate to severe MS can be found in Chapters 8 and 11.)

It should be emphasised that some people diagnosed with primary progressive MS may follow a milder course than that described above. It can be very distressing for them to read constantly that primary progressive MS is severe and relentless when their own experience is very different. It is unclear whether or not this is due to incorrect labelling of their MS as primary progressive or that they have a less severe form of primary progressive MS. Some people follow a very mild and largely unnoticed relapsing-remitting phase and are only diagnosed with MS as they reach the secondary progressive phase, which is likely to follow a correspondingly mild course. With no evident past history of problems there is no easy way at this stage, to differentiate between secondary progressive or primary progressive disease and some people may be wrongly ascribed to the primary progressive category (McDonnell and Hawkins, 1996).

Confirming a diagnosis of primary progressive MS can be very difficult. As can be seen below, primary progressive disease is very different from other types of MS and it is really only over time that a neurologist can be sure the individual has primary progressive disease. Diagnostic criteria have been proposed to assist in the diagnostic process (Thompson *et al.*, 2000). These criteria recommend that at least one year of clinical progression is documented prior to making a diagnosis of primary progressive MS. Three levels of diagnostic certainty are defined (i.e. definite, probable and possible) based on the clinical picture, cerebrospinal fluid analysis and magnetic resonance imaging. It is hoped that with further research to confirm these criteria, people with primary progressive MS can be diagnosed with certainty allowing them to access the necessary help, support and advice as soon as possible.

Progressive-relapsing MS

This is said to occur when someone experiences a progressive course from onset with clearly defined relapses superimposed. This type of MS is very rare and is included here for the sake of completion. There is a growing school of thought that this does not represent a different type of MS but is in fact a more extreme form of either primary progressive or secondary progressive MS (see Figure 3.1).

Is primary progressive MS a different disease?

There is an ongoing debate as to whether or not primary progressive MS actually constitutes a separate disease or whether it is just a more severe form of MS. The debate stems from the many differences between primary progressive and other types of MS, both in terms of the clinical course and the pathophysiology. The differences are as follows:

1. There is much less inflammation evident on MRI scans of the brain in primary progressive MS. However there are often multiple plaques evident in the spine (Revesz *et al.*, 1994).
2. It may take at least two years to confirm the diagnosis and rule out any recurrence of relapses (Thompson *et al.*, 1997).
3. Patients tend to present later with most people being at least 40 years old at diagnosis (Thompson *et al.*, 1997).

4. The normal male to female ratio in MS is 1:2; however, in primary progressive MS more males than females tend to develop the disease (Runmarker and Anderson, 1993).

5. Patients tend to experience fewer severe cognitive problems, possibly because of fewer lesions occurring in the brain (Vleugels *et al.*, 1998).

6. There are some immunological differences, including increased secretion of immunoglobulin G with less evidence of blood–brain barrier breakdown (Thompson *et al.*, 1997).

7. People with primary progressive MS are thought to suffer a greater degree of cerebral atrophy than in other types of MS, although the mechanism for this is not fully understood. This accounts in part for the steady deterioration experienced by people with primary progressive disease as opposed to the more common relapsing-remitting course (Stevenson *et al.*, 2000).

Despite these differences the evidence for primary progressive MS being a separate disease in its own right remains equivocal. There is not yet enough known about the pathological processes involved to be certain whether or not there is more than one disease which should be included under the heading of MS (McDonald and Thompson, 1997).

Benign MS

This is the mildest type of MS and the individual remains fully functional for at least 15 years after onset of the disease. It is likely that about 10% of people with MS follow a benign course. The long-term outlook for someone with benign disease is generally good but as always in MS there are exceptions and a few people with benign MS may go on to develop significant disability in later life.

The diagnosis of benign MS can only truly be made retrospectively. However, the term is sometimes used by clinicians to indicate mild disease. This can lead to confusion, as individuals who may only have been diagnosed with MS for a relatively short period of time believe they have benign MS; if their disease should subsequently follow a more severe course, they can find this difficult to reconcile with their original diagnosis.

Case study 3

CA presented with optic neuritis and pins and needles in her right hand and arm. She had had an episode of weakness in her right leg some months previously that had resolved spontaneously. C was diagnosed with MS based on her clinical history and the results of the neurological examination, lumbar puncture and MR scan. She was informed she had a benign form of MS.

During the next two years her condition unfortunately deteriorated. She developed significant visual defects and permanent weakness in her right leg, which meant that she had to walk with a stick. Fatigue also became an overwhelming problem and she was unable to walk far even with her stick. C began to use her wheelchair when out of the house more and more.

C became increasingly anxious and began to doubt her diagnosis. She could not understand why she should be having so many problems so soon after diagnosis when she had 'benign' MS. C became convinced that her symptoms were caused by something other then MS. When she saw the neurologist, she requested repeat MRI scans as she was convinced that she had a brain tumour.

It was only after considerable work with the neurologist, MS specialist nurse and psychologist that C accepted that her symptoms were all caused by MS and that unfortunately her MS was not benign in nature. Once she realised that her MS was a more progressive form, she was able to move forward and begin to accept the functional limitations she was living with.

Malignant or Marburg's MS

This is an extremely rare form of MS and is characterised by an acute onset with rapid decline in function culminating in death. It is such an atypical form that diagnosis is very difficult and treatments are largely ineffective. The implications for the patient, family and interdisciplinary team are very different than in other types of MS as it is effectively terminal.

It must be stressed that the vast majority of health care professionals will be unlikely ever to come across this type of MS. It is still rare enough to warrant single case reports in the medical journals (Bitsch *et al.*, 1999).

Practical problems in classifying an individual's MS

The type of MS an individual has is not usually immediately obvious and often only becomes apparent over time. However much of the available literature discusses the different types of MS in very black and white terms and as a result patients often become anxious to know what sort of

MS they have. Although on paper the different types appear to be very distinct, in reality the edges between the different types of MS are blurred and they may be better described as a continuum with different categories occurring at certain stages along the continuum.

Knowing what type of MS they are living with makes no real difference to the treatment or support offered to them. Indeed, informing someone of their type of MS (if known), may cause unnecessary concern and anxiety depending on the individual's understanding of the terms used. Care should be taken to explain that people with the same type of MS do not all reach the same level of disability. For example, as noted above, people diagnosed with primary progressive MS will not necessarily become severely disabled. If severe disability is going to occur this will often become evident within the first few years of onset. Similarly people who experience a relatively mild course over the first few years are less likely to develop severe disability later in life. Unfortunately there are always exceptions and each patient is different and each must be dealt with on an individual basis.

When talking about types of MS with patients and their families it is more useful to discuss individual prognostic indicators (see below) rather than focusing on which type of MS they have. NB: any discussion about prognosis should ideally be referred to the neurologist or MS specialist nurse. Prognosis in MS is best approached with a combination of caution and a crystal ball; it is still more of an art form than a science, although work to refine our understanding of prognostic indicators continues. The unpredictable nature of MS should be stressed to the patient and any indications of prognosis should be given in general terms.

Prognosis

The course of MS is so varied and unpredictable that it is impossible to provide individuals with any certain idea as to their future in terms of their disease. However some long-term studies on different populations have allowed us to develop some indicators of prognosis.

Table 3.1 lists some of the factors most commonly reported as being associated with a good or conversely, a worse prognosis (Leviæ *et al.*, 1999). Care should be taken when interpreting studies about prognosis as a literature search will usually reveal studies contradicting each other. This is not necessarily a reflection on the studies themselves but serves to illustrate the methodological difficulties inherent in studies of the natural history of MS. One of the main problems is establishing a database of

Table 3.1 Prognostic indicators in MS

Factors indicating a good prognosis:
- Female gender
- Sensory symptoms at onset
- Optic neuritis at onset
- Mild disability five years from onset
- Long intervals between attacks

Factors indicating a worse prognosis:
- Male gender
- Pyramidal or cerebellar signs at onset
- Multi-symptom onset
- Frequent attacks in first two years
- Moderate to severe impairment five years from onset

people with MS which is both complete and which contains long-term, regularly updated data.

Dr Weinshenker and colleagues have written a series of papers based on such a database from which we have been able to base much of our information regarding prognosis (Weinshenker *et al.*, 1998). There are other databases containing long-term data on specific populations such as the Danish MS registry, which was established in 1944 (Brønnum-Hansen *et al.*, 1994). More recently established databases such as NARCOMS (the North American Research Committee on MS) are also able to provide valuable natural history data and serve an increasingly important role in recruiting people for trials etc.

Unfortunately there is not yet anything on this scale in the UK or Europe although there are plans for something similar to be set up in the near future. It is likely, however, that the information gathered by the existing databases can be transposed to populations in the UK and Europe as the population of America and Canada is largely derived from migrants originating in Europe (Rudge, 1999).

Analysis of the databases has given us various prognostic indicators; for example, we now know that 50% of people with MS will reach an EDSS of 6.0 (i.e. needing a walking aid) within five years of disease onset while only 10% will become wheelchair bound in the same time period. It is also evident that an individual's level of disability (or ability) five years after the onset of their MS is strongly predictive of their future course (Weinshenker *et al.*, 1998).

The time when patients most need a guide as to what to expect with their MS is at diagnosis and often at a later time of changing needs, for example during a relapse or the transition phase between relapsing-remitting and secondary progressive MS.

Many people, be they newly diagnosed with MS or family and friends of people with MS, have preconceptions about the disease and what the diagnosis means.

For many this may be the image of an individual who quickly becomes wheelchair bound and is able to do little for themselves. As has been noted, this image is not an accurate one and this type of rapid progression is very rare. Almost half of people with MS are still enjoying a full and active life many years after diagnosis. The prognostic indicators described above can be used to explain to patients and their families that MS does not necessarily mean a wheelchair and can be used to provide some reassurance for most people with MS.

Measuring disability in MS

As can be seen from the preceding discussion about types of MS, the level of disability varies widely between different people irrespective of their type of MS.

Attempts to measure and define disability have been made over the years in many different ways and an overview of the different scales that have evolved specific to MS are included below.

An attempt to define the key terms associated with disability has been made by the World Health Organisation (cited in Wade, 1996).

Impairment: Loss or abnormality of psychological, physiological or anatomical structure or function.

Disability: Any restriction or lack of ability (resulting from an impairment) to perform an activity within the range considered normal for a human being.

Handicap: Any disadvantage for a given individual resulting from an impairment or disability that limits or prevents the fulfilment of a role that is normal for that individual.

One of the many difficulties inherent in measuring and defining disability is that it means different things to different people. People with MS, their partners and children, neurologists, interdisciplinary team members etc. will all focus on different aspects of an individual's disability. The WHO definitions attempt to bring together both the medical and social models of disability (see Box 3.1).

> **Box 3.1** A description of the medical and social models of disability
>
> Medical Model: Any difficulties in function an individual experiences are caused directly by their health problems.
>
> Social Model: Difficulties in function experienced by the individual are caused by the environment rather than the disease. For example an individual needing to use a wheelchair would be as mobile and independent as someone who can walk without assistance if there were no steps or kerbs, doorways were wide enough, appropriate floor surfaces were used everywhere, counter heights were low enough and other people's attitudes were the same as towards any other individual etc. etc.

These definitions and models of disability allow an identification and evaluation of needs to be made and ensure that we have a common language when discussing issues of research, health care resource allocation and the management of welfare resources etc. (Üstün and Leonardi, 1998).

Attempts to measure disability specific to MS have been going on for many years and there are a wide variety of rating scales available. Measures of disability in MS are necessary to define the care and support needed from the interdisciplinary team and the social changes needed to allow the individual to work etc. (Thompson and Hobart, 1998). They are also used extensively to measure improvements in specific areas for therapeutic or research purposes.

Rating scales

The scales used to measure disability are many and varied; some are better than others but none is perfect. They vary both in terms of the aspect of disability measured and in their relevance to the person with MS and the clinician.

The ideal requirements of any rating scale are listed in Table 3.2. At the present time there is no one scale which fulfils all these properties (and in truth there is unlikely to be, although it is hoped one can be developed that approximates to this ideal). Limitations are due in part to the problems inherent in studying MS. These include the variability of signs and symptoms which may be experienced, the unpredictability of the disease, its lifelong duration and the apparently poor correlation between pathology (as seen on MRI scans) and the signs and symptoms experienced by the individual. An overview of the more common scales follows.

Table 3.2 Requirements of the ideal rating scale in MS

- Relevant to both the clinician and the person with MS
- Sensitive to change
- Predictive of future course
- Disease specific
- Cost-effective
- Easy to use
- Multi-dimensional
- Good inter-rater reliability
- Reproducible
- Sensitive to the full range of impairments

Source: After Amato and Ponziani 1999; Frederikson *et al.*, 1996.

Expanded Disability Status Scale (EDSS)

This is currently the most frequently used rating scale in MS. It can only be administered by a neurologist or trained clinician and is heavily biased towards problems with mobility. It takes little account of upper limb problems, cognition, fatigue etc. The patient is scored from 0 to 10, 0 representing someone with no impairments and 10 representing death from MS and the scale moves up in half points. It is an ordinal scale, which means that each point on the scale cannot be compared to any other in terms of progression or the degree of change in disability represented. People spend more time around scores 1–2 and 6–7 than at other points on the scale (Frederikson *et al.*, 1996). As a result of this the scale is not very sensitive and does not highlight changes that may be significant to the patient. The main points of the scale are listed below (Kurtzke, 1983).

0–3.5	Patient exhibits neurological signs rather than evident impairments
4–5.5	Patient develops increasing difficulty with walking over progressively shorter distances
6	Patient requires a stick/crutch to walk 100 yards
6.5	Patient requires 2 sticks to walk 20 yards
7–8	Patient is restricted to a wheelchair
8.5–9.5	Patient is bed-bound and increasingly dependent for all their needs
10	Death due to MS

Despite these difficulties the EDSS remains the 'tarnished gold standard' of scales at the present time (Thompson and Hobart, 1998). Different therapeutic trials have used progression as measured by the EDSS as an outcome measure, particularly in trials looking at the effects of interferons on MS (PRISMS Study Group, 1998; INFB Multiple Sclerosis Study Group, 1993). It has been found that the reliability of the EDSS can be improved by using the same assessing clinician throughout, using standardised documentation and protocols for the neurological examination with definitions for specific terms included (Frederikson *et al.*, 1996).

Scripps Neurological Rating Scale (NRS)

The Scripps Neurological Rating Scale (Sipe *et al.*, 1984) has been used in many trials. It is largely based on the findings of the neurological examination with additional categories for bladder, bowel and sexual problems. Someone with no impairments scores 100. Unfortunately the scale can be difficult to apply as clear guidelines are not available and data concerning validity and severity are somewhat thin on the ground.

Other scales in use include the Barthel Index (Mahoney and Barthel, 1965) and the Functional Independence Measure (FIM) among others. These measures are not disease specific and the nurse is most likely to come across them in the context of therapy interventions or rehabilitation. The Barthel is relatively simple to use but neglects to take account of any difficulties the patient may experience with cognition or communication. As a result the FIM and FIM/FAM were developed as an extension of the Barthel. It has been shown, however, that these scales, which require lengthy training to use, are no more reliable or responsive than the Barthel. However all these scales are more responsive than the EDSS (Thompson and Hobart, 1998).

The patients' perspective

The scales mentioned above are all concerned with measuring physical disability. It is becoming recognised that the medical model, which these scales are based on, is not usually the most appropriate from the point of view of the person with MS. People themselves are more concerned with issues related to quality of life such as fatigue and mental health whereas clinicians are more likely to focus on mobility (Rothwell *et al.*, 1997).

Dr van Overstaten, a GP with MS, describes very vividly what scoring in MS means to him on a personal level. He states

> I score myself all the time. On a short term basis several times a day to foresee problems in the coming hours and to assess if I have to call for help for the duties I have to perform. This scoring is done on a very subtle level, even the most minute changes of lifting power in my legs can mean the difference between tripping over my shadow or sliding over it. (van Overstaten, 1999)

He goes on to say

> In the long-term I score myself on recurring activities throughout the year. Every
> year for example a friend of mine invites me to join him on a sailing expedition, a
> tricky activity for someone with diminished strength and sense of balance; and
> although I always feel very happy being able to join him, it does make one acutely
> aware of the amount of deterioration that progresses steadily through the year.
> On the other hand, the number of voluntary activities ... put the degree of
> disability or better, the degree of ability in a different, perhaps more favourable
> perspective.

Dr van Overstaten shows us that what matters to patients is their ability
to meet their daily work, family and social commitments with minimal
help from others; this ability does not necessarily depend on mobility.

Neurological rating scales are constantly being developed and refined
and the factors relevant to patients are being taken more into account.

Guy's Neurological Disability Scale

The Guy's Neurological Disability Scale (Sharrack and Hughes, 1999)
was devised in response to the difficulties apparent in the scales described
above. The scale is user friendly, reported as being acceptable to patients
as well as neurologists and can be applied by any health care professional.
It has 12 separate categories including cognition, mood, sexual function
and fatigue. Preliminary work shows the scale to be valid, reliable and
responsive although further independent study is needed to confirm this.

There are many other rating scales in use and it is beyond the scope of
this book to describe them all. It should be remembered that it is unlikely
a scale will ever be devised that fully meets all the requirements in Table
3.2. However the majority of scales available do allow us to make some
valid measurements and comparisons. Clinicians are now realising that it
is likely a number of different scales should be used to provide a comprehensive measure of the impact of an individual's disability on themselves
and their lives.

CHAPTER 4

Disease modifying therapies

Introduction

Approximately 85% of people have relapsing-remitting disease when they first develop MS. The majority of these people will go on to develop secondary progressive MS within 10–15 years of disease onset. While there are many treatments and therapies available to enable symptomatic relief, it is only in the last few years that any treatment proven to affect the actual course of MS has been developed.

Interferon beta 1b (Betaferon) was the first disease modifying therapy to be licensed in the UK in 1995. This was followed by Avonex in 1997 and Rebif in 1998, both Avonex and Rebif are interferon beta 1a compounds. Most recently, Copaxone (glatiramer acetate previously known as Copolymer 1) was licensed in the UK in 2000. These treatments have all been proven to be effective in reducing the number of relapses an individual experiences and in ensuring that any continuing relapses are less severe and of shorter duration than previously experienced.

However the disease modifying treatments have been dogged by controversy since their launch and the controversy is ongoing at the time of writing. The theory and practice of using beta interferons and glatiramer acetate is examined below and some of the reasons for the controversy are explored in more depth.

What are interferons?

Interferons occur naturally in the body as a component of the immune system. There are three different types of interferon: gamma interferon, beta interferon and alpha interferon. It is known that gamma interferon causes an inflammatory response resulting in an increased frequency of exacerbations or relapses (Panitch *et al.*, 1987). However, alpha interferon and beta interferon work by damping down the immune response so having the effect of lessening the inflammation, which is responsible for much of the damage in MS.

Glatiramer acetate is not found naturally within the body, it is in fact a synthetic protein, made up of a mixture of amino acids, which resembles myelin.

Trial design and unanswered questions

While the trial designs for the three beta interferons now commercially available have a number of similarities, there are also some important differences between them. The different approach taken by the different pharmaceutical companies has, at least in part, contributed somewhat to the controversy and lack of clarity surrounding the different products. This said, in relapsing-remitting MS, all three have been proven to reduce the number of relapses a suitable individual experiences by about a third and any relapses that people do still experience are shorter and less severe while on treatment.

All of the trials were multi-centre and placebo controlled in design. This means that participants were each allocated to either a treatment or a placebo group and neither the clinician nor the participant knew which group they had been allocated to. The participants were then closely monitored for the duration of their time in the trial.

People recruited into the initial trials all had a confirmed diagnosis of MS and were known to be experiencing fairly frequent relapses. However, one factor which makes it difficult to compare and interpret the different trial results as a whole is that each trial recruited people with differing levels of disability:

Betaferon	EDSS 0.0–5.5	at least 2 relapses in previous 2 years (INFB MS Study Group, 1993)
Avonex	EDSS 0.0–3.5	at least 2 relapses in previous 3 years (Jacobs *et al.*, 1996)
Rebif	EDSS 0.0–5.0	at least 2 relapses in previous 2 years (PRISMS Study Group, 1998)

It should be remembered that the EDSS (i.e. Expanded Disability Status Scale) is a relatively insensitive measure of disability although it is widely recognised and accepted as the best available, certainly at the time the trials were designed and implemented. In crude terms, the higher the EDSS level, the more disabled an individual is. Thus it can be seen that participants on the Avonex trial were much less disabled with less active disease than those on either the Betaferon or Rebif trials. This makes direct comparison of results problematical.

All the trials demonstrated a statistically significant reduction in the number of relapses experienced. However, because of the different trial designs, direct comparison, even of specific results, is difficult. For example, the Betaferon trial demonstrated an overall reduction in relapse rate of about 34% while the Avonex trial demonstrated only an 18% reduction overall (ABN, 2001). However, the researchers state that the true figure is nearer 32%. As the recruitment for the Avonex trial was staggered over a prolonged period, if data from a two-year time interval is analysed, some individuals on the trial will only have been using Avonex for a short time. If, however, the data from all individuals who have been taking Avonex (or placebo) for two years is analysed then the figure for reduction in relapse rate is nearer 32% (Herndon, 2000). The numbers of people who have dropped out of the trial before the two-year time period are also disregarded when calculating the figure of 32%. To complicate matters further, the Rebif trial used two different doses, using the lower dose of 22 micrograms showed a reduction in relapse rate of 27%. The higher dose of 44 micrograms showed a reduction of 33% (PRISMS Study Group, 1998).

There are also many other difficulties surrounding the trials that have resulted in an ongoing debate surrounding the relative efficacy of the beta interferons.

The effect of glatiramer acetate was also studied using a multi-centred, placebo controlled trial design (Johnson et al., 1995). Participants needed to have a confirmed diagnosis of MS, be aged 18–45 with an EDSS of 0.0–5.0. The primary end-point of the trial was reduction in relapse rate. The trial ran for two years and the rate of relapse was found to be reduced by about 29%. Copaxone has not been central to the debate surrounding the beta interferons; this is due in part to its being a totally different product, therefore making direct comparisons difficult and also, primarily, because it has only recently been licensed in the UK.

The beta interferons have also been examined to determine their effect on the number of demyelinating lesions seen on MR (magnetic resonance) scans. All three demonstrated a significant reduction in lesion load as measured on MR scans. Copaxone trials did not include large-scale MRI studies although more recent trials have shown a reduction in lesion load (Comi, Fillipi for the Copaxone Study Group, 1999).

There is also much debate ongoing as to the effect of beta interferon on disease progression in people with secondary progressive disease. A study of people with secondary progressive MS taking Betaferon (European Study Group, 1998) did demonstrate a statistically significant slowing in the rate of progression. As a result of this trial Betaferon is now licensed for use in people who have secondary progressive MS. However, a study of patients on Rebif failed to demonstrate any significant slowing in the progression of disability (SPECTRIMS, 2000). This has led to some uncertainty as to the effectiveness of beta interferon in this context and further work is needed to clarify this point.

In practice, many people with MS who are on interferon or glatiramer acetate have noted a reduction in relapse rate of at least one-third and in some cases have experienced virtually no relapses at all (unpublished audit data). Although disease-modifying therapies don't suit everyone, most people find that in addition to a reduction in relapse rate, they are generally more stable with less 'bad days'. Many individuals also find that the treatments have a positive effect on their lives. There have been studies that have tried to quantify this in terms of cost (Parkin *et al.*, 1998; Forbes *et al.*, 1999). These studies have all demonstrated a disproportionately high cost per quality of life year gained (QALY). The cost per QALY has been put as high as £1,024,667 in the first study cited. However, in any such study it is vital that quality of life measures with relevance to the person with MS and not just the clinician are used. It is also essential that the cost analysis be made over the long term, i.e. 15–25 years and not just the next five. It is in the long term that any cost benefits are likely to become evident. A selection of comments from people taking Betaferon is shown in Figure 4.1. These illustrate the positive effect beta interferon can have for people with MS.

Despite the demonstrable effect on relapse rate, reduction in disease activity as shown on MR scans and the positive responses of many people using beta interferon, many health authorities and the vast majority of health boards in Scotland have refused to fund the prescribing of disease modifying therapies. Some health authorities have funded only a small number of individuals regardless of the amount of need. This is due to a number of factors including the ongoing debates surrounding trial design

- 'After only a few weeks on the Betaferon I became more upright in my walking with a lot more stamina.'
- ' I was experiencing a relapse every 2–3 months, with Betaferon it has been six months between relapses.'
- 'My stamina has returned to near normal. Previously affected limbs have regained their strength.'
- 'Side-effects definitely subside.'
- 'I am a little worse but the way I think, if I hadn't taken it I could have been a lot worse.'
- 'If there is a chance of halting the effects of MS, a few red blotches are worth putting up with.'
- 'Normal symptoms have improved, pain and discomfort suppressed but severe relapses don't seem to be helped to any degree.'

Source: Burgess, 1998.

Figure 4.1 Examples of comments made by people taking Betaferon.

and lack of comparability between trials. Apart from these considerations cost is also a major factor. Beta interferons are priced at an average cost of about £10,000 per person per year while glatiramer acetate has been launched at a price of approximately £6,600 per person per year.

A number of questions remain unanswered and clarification of these points will be sought over the next few years.

- What are the long-term effects of using beta interferon and glatiramer acetate over 15–20 years?
- What is the effect on progression of disability in people with secondary progressive disease?
- How cost-effective are the treatments in the long term?
- What are the effects of disease modifying therapies on symptoms most relevant to individuals with MS, e.g. fatigue and cognition?

The different responses by the health authorities and health boards have resulted in a situation known as 'post code prescribing', i.e. the availability of disease modifying therapies for suitable individuals depends almost solely upon where that individual lives.

This situation is eminently unfair and perpetuates inequality of prescribing. In an attempt to resolve these problems the National Institute for Clinical Excellence (NICE) was asked to issue guidance on the use of beta interferon and glatiramer acetate.

NICE began their review and consultation process in August 1999. They issued a final appraisal determination in June 2000. These guidelines recommended that beta interferons should not be prescribed for any more individuals with MS although existing patients could remain on treatment. This decision was greeted with dismay by patients, health professionals and pharmaceutical companies alike. All interested parties, including the Association of British Neurologists (ABN) and MS specialist nurses (coordinated by the RCN), lodged an appeal. As a result of the evidence submitted at the appeal, the guidance issued in June 2000 was withdrawn. At the time of writing it is expected that further guidance will be issued in the second half of 2001 (Scott, 2000).

Practicalities of using disease modifying therapies

Who should be prescribed beta interferon or glatiramer acetate?

Interferon betas and glatiramer acetate are only helpful for a small proportion of people with MS (approximately 7%). At present, the ABN guidelines state that the individual must have confirmed MS, must be able to walk approximately 100m independently and have had at least two confirmed relapses in the previous two years (ABN, 2001). In effect people must be ambulant and have active disease. Betaferon is the only disease modifying therapy licensed for use in people with secondary progressive MS and people in this category must also be ambulant over at least 10m and have had at least two disabling relapses in the last two years. The ABN only recommends the use of Betaferon in secondary progressive patients who are also having relapses. These guidelines may change depending on the outcome of the NICE appraisal.

Using interferon

A neurologist must prescribe beta interferon or glatiramer acetate and most centres will hold specialist clinics to assess and monitor patients on disease modifying therapies. The MS specialist nurse is also usually in attendance at these clinics as part of their role is to teach, support and monitor people using interferon.

Patients are referred to the prescribing neurologist and assessed with regard to disease type, relapse activity (i.e. two or more relapses in the last two years) and mobility.

Once a patient is assessed as suitable for treatment and the choice of disease modifying therapy has been made, the patient sees the MS specialist nurse. The MS nurse will then do a nursing assessment and discuss any issues outstanding regarding starting on treatment. The neurologist will request some blood tests to be taken prior to starting treatment. These are necessary as the blood levels of certain liver enzymes and the white cell count can be adversely affected by beta interferon. Glatiramer acetate does not affect blood levels and so individuals using this drug do not need routine blood tests. It is also important to ensure that if the patient is female she is not pregnant as neither beta interferon nor glatiramer acetate can be taken by anyone who may be pregnant as its safety in this context is unknown. It is thought that they may be abortigenic, i.e. they can cause a miscarriage. A pregnancy test may be necessary.

The ABN Guidelines also recommend that a protein electrophoresis test be conducted prior to starting treatment. This is in order to ensure that patients do not have a monoclonal gammopathy. (If interferons are given to someone with a monoclonal gammopathy, it can be fatal.)

It is also important to explain fully to patients and their partners the pros and cons of treatment and what they should expect in terms of both side effects and benefits. Many patients assessed for disease modifying therapy have unrealistic expectations which can adversely affect their compliance and, when unfulfilled, may contribute to feelings of depression.

Patients with their partners or a close friend are then asked to attend a training session where the MS specialist nurse will teach them how to prepare the injection and discuss the procedure for self-injection and management of side effects. If using Betaferon, Rebif or Copaxone the injection sites should be rotated and patient manuals are provided describing these. Suitable sites for injection include the front thighs, upper arms, buttocks and belly. Avonex is given by intra-muscular (IM) injection and can be given in the arm or buttock as is common for most IM injections.

Patients are then given an appointment for their first injection, which must be given in a hospital setting.

Once the first injection is given the MS nurse will assess the subsequent support needed to allow the patient to manage the injections themselves. Patients using Avonex will usually need to be given the injection by either their practice nurse or district nurse. However a few people are able to manage this themselves.

Once patients are established on treatment they must be seen regularly and at least every three months for the first 12 months and no less than six monthly for the duration of their time on treatment. At each appointment, any difficulties and side effects should be noted and appropriate advice given. The blood tests (see Table 4.1) should be repeated every three months for the first year of treatment; if these are normal then they need only be repeated six monthly thereafter. Any abnormal results should be acted upon accordingly as described below.

Table 4.1 Routine blood tests required when monitoring individuals using beta interferon

- Full blood count
- Urea and electrolytes (Us and Es)
- Liver function tests (including ALT/AST)
- GGT

Comparison of disease modifying therapies

As noted above, the four types of treatment that are available all have many similarities and differences. Table 4.2 compares the different types.

Management of side effects

Beta interferon

All of the interferons cause side effects and it is fair to say that the majority of people starting treatment will experience side effects to some degree although these normally wear off over time.

When first starting treatment the most common side effects are flu-like symptoms and problems at the injection site. The flu-like symptoms vary from person to person, they may be mild with just a slight increase in fatigue or be much more severe, presenting with shivering, aches and a general feeling of being unwell. These symptoms normally occur within 2–5 hours of the injection and with Betaferon or Rebif the side effects wear off approximately 10–12 hours after onset. People using Avonex may find that the symptoms last longer, i.e. 24–48 hours initially. These flu-like symptoms may also include headaches, fatigue, fever and muscle aches (Lublin *et al.*, 1996).

Table 4.2 A comparison of beta interferons and glatiramer acetate

Trade name	Avonex	Betaferon	Rebif	Copaxone
Generic name	Interferon beta 1a	Interferon beta 1b	Interferon beta 1a	Glatiramer acetate
Storage temperature	< 25°C	2–8°C	2–8°C	2–8°C
Administered	Intra-muscular, once weekly	Subcutaneously, alternate days	Subcutaneously, 3x weekly	Subcutaneously, daily
Presentation	Syringe with pre-filled diluent	Syringe with pre-filled diluent	Syringe pre-filled with active drug	Diluent and powder separate
Dose per ml diluent	30mcg	8 miu	22mcg/44mcg	20mg
Licensed for relapsing-remitting patients	Yes	Yes	Yes	Yes
Licensed for secondary progressive patients	No	Yes	No	No
Reduction in relapse rate (ABN, 2001)	18% (32% – see text)	34%	22mcg – 27% 44mcg – 33%	29%
MRI data (ABN, 2001)	50% reduction in enhancing lesions	70% reduction in enhancing lesions	70% reduction in enhancing lesions	35% reduction in enhancing lesions (Preliminary results – studies ongoing)
EDSS of patients in trial	0-3.5	0-5.5	0-5.0	0-5.0

These flu-like symptoms should wear off after about three months. In practice many people find that the worst effects have subsided after 2–3 injections and by 4–6 weeks have almost gone. In order to minimise any problems, patients are encouraged to take an analgesic such as paracetamol or brufen soon after the injection and for up to 24 hours afterwards as needed. By taking the injection at night patients also find they are able to sleep through the worst of the symptoms and this can make the first few weeks of treatment much more bearable.

Very occasionally people may also find that their MS becomes much worse for a few hours. This tends to affect the individual's weakest point, e.g. if they have a lot of visual problems, their vision may be affected or if their mobility is poor they may find they are unable to walk or even stand. Understandably this can be extremely frightening for the individual and their family; however, the MS nurse should reassure the individual that if this happens it passes within a few hours and usually only happens on the first injection, and then only rarely.

Glatiramer acetate

The side-effect profile of glatiramer acetate is somewhat different than for beta interferon. It is generally much better tolerated than the interferons although approximately 15% of people will experience some transitory chest pain or tightness accompanied by anxiety, flushing, sweating and sometimes a perceived difficulty in breathing. These symptoms can understandably be frightening for both patient and nurse! However, it is thought that the symptoms are largely benign (Hawkins and Wolinsky, 2000). The side effects only last for a short time (about 30 minutes) and resolve spontaneously; they may recur sporadically for a susceptible individual. Good education and full explanations of what to expect on starting treatment before the first injection is given will help the patient cope more easily with the side effects.

Injection site reactions

Injection site reactions can occur with the subcutaneous injections. Betaferon and Rebif can cause people to develop a red mark at the site, which fades over a period of weeks. Occasionally the injection site becomes painful and hardened red lumps can form which may take some time to ease. The use of a mild, topical steroid cream can help reduce the reaction if severe. Very occasionally people develop necrosis at the site of a particular injection (only 1–2% people experience this); this may be the result of poor technique but is more often due to a particular susceptibility in that individual. Should the skin become broken at any injection site, the individual should discontinue treatment and contact their MS specialist nurse or GP immediately. Copaxone can also cause problems at the injection site, causing pain, reddening and, potentially, hardening of the skin in the area of the injection. This usually subsides relatively quickly. There is no evidence of any skin necrosis occurring in people using glatiramer acetate.

Other common side effects are listed in Table 4.3. As noted above, most patients cope very well with the side effects and a few may well experience no side effects at all. A self-report survey of patients in the early stages of treatment indicated that the majority of people described the side effects as no worse than 'a little uncomfortable' (Burgess, 1998).

Table 4.3 Commonly experienced side effects of beta interferons

- Fatigue
- Stiffness
- Night sweats
- Insomnia
- Altered menstrual cycle
- Depression
- Low white blood cell count
- Raised liver function tests
- Headaches
- Weakness

Depression and interferons

In the trial of Betaferon (INFB MS Study Group, 1993) there were a few patients taking Betaferon, as opposed to placebo, who became very depressed and experienced ideas of suicide. One individual actually committed suicide. Understandably this caused a great deal of concern and there were fears that Betaferon and by proxy the other interferons could have a direct effect on mood in some individuals causing severe depression.

Whether or not depression is a direct result of taking interferon continues to be debated although it is coming to be thought much less likely that there is a direct link (Borràs et al., 1999). It should be noted that as part of the protocol for the original trial, patients were not allowed to take any analgesics etc. which patients are now encouraged to take to moderate the side effects of treatment. There was also no support offered to individuals during the trial by nurses or other health care professionals. It should also be noted that neither the secondary progressive trial of Betaferon nor the trials of Avonex or Rebif showed any evidence of an increase in depression or suicidal thoughts compared with patients on placebo. The incidence of depression reported in patients prescribed Betaferon as a licensed medication varies from 4% (Lublin et al., 1996) to 41% (Mohr et al., 1997).

It is most likely that any link between depression and interferon is an indirect consequence of taking the medication. As well as coping with the MS and the effect this has on their lives, patients are suddenly faced with frequent injections that initially may make them feel worse. Patients also find that, particularly if using denial as a coping mechanism, being faced with a box of injections for their MS every time they open the fridge door can be difficult to cope with. It should also be remembered that people with MS are just as likely to be depressed as any one else due to problems with family/work/finance etc.

Before starting treatment, patients and their partners or family should be warned that depression might occur but that they should not expect to feel depressed. If they do, they should be advised to contact their MS specialist nurse or GP as soon as possible so that appropriate action can be taken. Appropriate treatment of any depression with counselling and/or anti-depressants can be very effective and helpful in assisting patients to comply with their treatment regime (Mohr et al., 1997).

Troubleshooting

Included below is a list of the more common problems that an individual may be faced with when using disease modifying therapies. Most problems can be easily solved and if they persist, the patient or other health care professional working with them should contact the MS specialist nurse or the neurologist.

Pain/red lumps at injection site

Creams can help, e.g. E45, witch hazel or mild steroid cream. The MS nurse should review the patient's technique and ensure that the injection site is rotated. The use of aids such as an autoject device should be considered.

Bruising at injection site

Bruising generally occurs as a result of hitting a capillary while injecting, however some areas do seem to mark more readily than others, simply changing the injection site may relieve the problem.

Necrosis at injection site

This is a serious complication and the interferon must be stopped immediately until the site has healed. The patient may require antibiotics to clear any secondary infection. Treatment can be recommenced in other injection sites once the necrotic area has healed.

Flu-like symptoms won't settle

The patient may benefit from a drug holiday, alternatively, titration of the dose can be helpful. If all else fails, discontinuation of treatment should be considered.

Insomnia

Changing the injection time to earlier in the day, with appropriate analgesic cover, can be very helpful.

Weakness within a few hours of injection

The patient should be advised to contact their MS nurse, the problem will usually wear off after 1 or 2 injections – if not the patient may need to discontinue treatment.

Low white blood cell count

If this is below normal but greater than $3.0 \times 10^9/L$ then the individual should be able to continue on treatment. Bloods should be repeated every 4–6 weeks until the levels are back to normal. If the white blood cell count is less than $3.0 \times 10^9/L$, treatment should be stopped and can be recommenced once the levels have returned to normal.

Increased liver function tests (LFTs)

If the aminotransferases (ALT or AST) or gamma-glutamyl transpeptidase (GGT) are elevated by more than 5–10 times the normal level then treatment should be stopped and recommenced once levels have returned to an acceptable reading.

Low haemoglobin

This is rarely a direct effect of treatment and should be investigated and treated as required.

Pregnancy

The patient must stop interferon or glatiramer acetate immediately.

Breast-feeding

Patients must be advised not to breast-feed while taking beta interferon or glatiramer acetate.

Depression

Depending on the cause and severity, counselling and/or anti-depressants may be required. A drug holiday may be helpful.

Relapse

The need for treatment, if a relapse occurs, should be assessed by the neurologist in the same way as for patients who are not on any disease modifying therapy; steroids can be administered if required and interferon treatment is normally continued.

Drug interactions

Beta interferon and glatiramer acetate have very few interactions with other medications and people can still take any other medication, including antibiotics, as required.

Patients and their families are given a contact number (usually that of the MS nurse) and are encouraged to phone if they have any concerns. If the patient has any difficulties while on treatment the nurse will liaise with the neurologist and an appropriate course of action will be taken.

The above list of potential problems and suggested solutions is intended as a guide only. Each neurologist will work in a slightly different way and patients experiencing problems should be encouraged to contact their MS nurse.

If all else fails

Some patients are not able to tolerate a particular type of disease modifying therapy. They may experience unremitting flu-like symptoms or develop blood abnormalities that refuse to settle or their MS may continue to deteriorate. If this occurs and attempts to resolve the problems meet with no success then it may be necessary to stop treatment. Patients may sometimes tolerate one type of therapy where they do not tolerate another.

Interferon beta and glatiramer acetate are not helpful for everyone; each patient must be assessed individually and in discussion with the neurologist, MS nurse and themselves. If a patient is unable to tolerate a particular type of therapy it may be worth considering an alternative disease modifying therapy; other options are described below.

Stopping disease modifying therapies

Some people may have to stop treatment due to intolerable side effects or if a pregnancy is planned. Treatment should also be stopped if it ceases to be effective. The ABN guidelines (2001) state that if an individual experiences two or more confirmed, disabling relapses within 12 months, or the individual develops secondary progressive MS, or they become unable to walk with or without assistance for at least 6 months, then treatment should be stopped. Patients should be reviewed formally every two years.

There is no rebound effect on stopping treatment and patients can stop immediately they are advised so to do without fear of any resulting problems.

Neutralising antibodies

It is known that in some patients antibodies develop to the interferon; these are known as neutralising antibodies or NABs. They were originally thought to cancel out the effect of the interferon. However, careful studies have since shown that patients have a variable antibody status and can switch between having and not having antibodies regardless of interferon treatment. It has also been shown that the presence of NABs does not cause any increase in relapse rate as would be expected if they prevented the interferon from working (Petkau and White, 1997). Any decision to stop treatment should be a clinical one and not based on the presence or absence of NABs. The clinical importance of NABs continues to be debated (Arnason and Dianzani, 1998).

Immunoglobulin

Intravenous immunoglobulin has been used to treat various neurological diseases such as Guillain-Barré syndrome and other neuropathies for some time. More recently attention has turned to exploring its effectiveness against MS.

Various trials have been conducted, each focusing on a different effect of the immunoglobulin on MS, i.e. relapse rate (Achiron *et al.*, 1998), disease progression (Fazekas *et al.*, 1997) and effect on lesion load on MRI scans (Sørensen *et al.*, 1998).

Overall results of these and other trials show a modest effect on slowing down disease progression, a significant reduction in relapse rate (at least equal to that achieved by beta interferon) and lesion load as seen on magnetic resonance scans.

Immunoglobulin is given by intravenous infusion once monthly. A bolus dose over five days may be given when starting treatment. The most effective dose and treatment regime in MS has yet to be formally researched, however the recommended dose is usually around 0.15–0.2g/Kg body weight (Fazekas *et al.*, 1999).

Immunoglobulin is usually well tolerated. The most commonly reported side effects are headaches and nausea. Should these occur they could be easily controlled with analgesics and anti-emetics; slowing down the rate of infusion may also help.

Overall immunoglobulin appears to offer an equally effective and well-tolerated alternative to beta interferon or glatiramer acetate. The costs of the drug including the costs of administration are high but significantly cheaper than beta interferon or glatiramer acetate. Further large-scale studies are needed to determine the most effective dose and examine the effects specific to MS.

As with beta interferon and glatiramer acetate, immunoglobulin is only effective for people with relapsing-remitting disease or patients with secondary progressive disease who are active and relatively mobile.

Mitoxantrone

This was originally developed to treat cancer but has recently been shown to reduce relapse rate, slow progression of disability and reduce lesion load on MRI scans in people with MS (Noseworthy *et al.*, 1999). It is unique in that it is also effective for some people with primary progressive MS. It is most often used as a rescue remedy for people who are deteriorating rapidly and who have not responded to other disease modifying treatments. Its use is not widespread at present and tends to be confined to specialist centres.

It is given by intravenous infusion and is relatively well tolerated. It is usually administered monthly for the first three months and then given once every three months for a specified course of treatment.

Mitoxantrone is bright blue in colour and turns urine blue/green; occasionally the sclera of the eyes may also take on a bluish tint. The main side effects tend to be fatigue and nausea; some people also experience hair loss. The nausea can be controlled with anti-emetic medication.

Summary

Many other therapies and combinations of therapies are being studied. At present the majority of treatments are for people with relapsing-remitting disease; however, trials with therapies in other categories of MS are ongoing. As we understand more about the pathogenesis of the different types of MS, further therapies will suggest themselves and be developed. In the meantime improved symptomatic treatment will help to maintain a better quality of life for people with MS while patients are waiting for further developments in the field of disease modifying therapies.

CHAPTER 5

Symptoms and their treatments

Functional anatomy of the central nervous system related to the signs and symptoms of MS

MS lesions are found in the brain and spine; the myelin sheath that facilitates transmission of impulses along the axons is damaged by an auto immune reaction (see Chapter 1). This results in the impulses becoming delayed or blocked completely, so resulting in the myriad of symptoms which may be experienced by the individual with MS. The particular signs and symptoms depend to some extent on the site of the lesion within the central nervous system; to this end a brief overview of the anatomy of the brain and spine follows.

The brain is composed of a number of different sections and is continuous with the spinal cord. The section linking the brain and spine is called the brain stem. The brain stem consists of three sections, the medulla oblongata, the pons and the midbrain. The medulla oblongata is continuous with the spinal cord and contains vital centres, i.e. the cardiac, respiratory and vasomotor centres. The medulla also controls some non-vital reflexes such as coughing, vomiting and swallowing.

The pons is situated above the medulla and helps to regulate respiration, the 5th, 6th, 7th and 8th cranial nerves exit here. The midbrain controls some aspects of hearing, vision and movement. The 3rd and 4th cranial nerves exit from the midbrain.

The cerebellum is the second largest part of the brain and lies below and partly covered by the cerebrum. The cerebellum is divided into two halves known as the cerebellar hemispheres. The outermost portion of the hemispheres is made up of grey matter (i.e. cell bodies) while the innermost portion is made up of white matter (i.e. axons). The cerebellum acts in conjunction with the cerebral cortex to produce skilled movements by co-ordinating muscles. The cerebellum is also responsible for maintaining an individual's equilibrium and balance. Thus cerebellar dysfunction may result in ataxia, tremor, balance and gait disturbances among others.

The diencephalon is located between the cerebrum and the midbrain and consists of four sections, the most important of which are the thalamus and hypothalamus. The thalamus acts as the main relay station for sensory impulses travelling to the cerebral cortex from the peripheral nerves. The thalamus allows an individual to make a crude recognition of sensations and is responsible for relaying sensory signals to other parts of the brain for 'fine tuning'. The thalamus is also responsible in part for reflex actions triggered by sensation, e.g. moving your hand away quickly from a painful stimulus.

The hypothalamus provides a link between the nervous system and the endocrine system. It also regulates an individual's appetite, body temperature and waking state and is responsible for some hormone production.

The cerebrum is divided into two halves known as the right and left cerebral hemispheres. Each hemisphere consists of five different lobes separated from each other by shallow grooves known as fissures or sulci. The surface of the cerebral hemispheres is convoluted; the convolutions are known as gyri (singular is gyrus). Each lobe is named after the skull bone beneath which it lies. The outer part of the cerebral hemispheres is made up of grey matter, while the inner part consists of white matter. Within the white matter the axons tend to be arranged to form tracts which circumvent the ventricles and form the roof of the lateral ventricles. They can be thought of as bundles of wires transferring impulses from one part of the brain to another. These white matter tracts are particularly prone to plaques caused by MS.

The complete understanding of the function of the cerebrum is not known. However it is known that the right and left hemispheres both operate with a different emphasis. The left side is normally responsible for language skills and controlled hand movements (remember the left side of the cerebrum controls the right side of the body and vice versa). The right side co-ordinates the perception of auditory non-speech stimuli as well as tactual and spatial relationships. The speech centres are usually in the left hemisphere, although approximately 10% of the population will have their speech centre in the right side or both. The frontal, parietal and temporal lobes all contain different aspects of speech control.

Memory is also co-ordinated within the cerebral cortex and particularly within the temporal, parietal and occipital lobes. Emotions are controlled via the limbic system, which is composed of a number of structures around the corpus callosum. Figure 5.1 illustrates the main structures of the brain.

Spinal cord

The spinal cord is continuous with the medulla oblongata of the brain stem and consists of 31 bilaterally paired spinal nerves.

    8 cervical (C 1-8)
    12 Thoracic (T 1-12)
    5 Lumbar (L1-5)
    5 Sacral (S1-5)
    1 Coccygeal

The centre of the spinal cord consists of grey matter, which is in turn surrounded by white matter made up of ascending and descending nerve fibres running between the brain and the appropriate spinal nerves. The ascending tracts carry impulses from peripheral nerves to relevant receptors

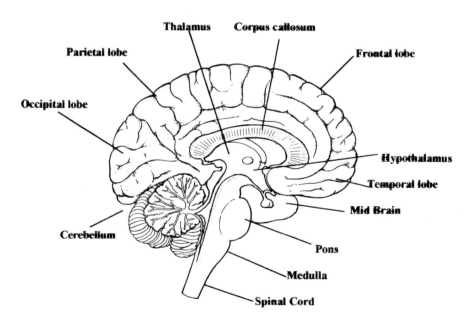

Figure 5.1 Diagram of the brain showing the main structures.

in the brain, e.g. pain, temperature, muscle and joint proprioception. Descending tracts originate from the cerebral cortex and brain stem and control movement, reflexes, muscle tone etc.

C1-4	Control sensation in the back of the head, front of the neck and the upper part of the shoulder. They also control the motor function of neck muscles
C5-8	Controls the diaphragm, arm and hand, also motor and some sensory function in scapula
T1-12	Chest and respiratory muscles
L1-5	Sensory perception and motor function of abdominal wall, genitalia, legs and buttocks

Cranial nerves

The 12 pairs of cranial nerves originate from the under surface of the brain, mostly from the brain stem. They are peripheral nerves and so are not affected directly by breakdown of their myelin sheath as MS only affects nerves in the central nervous system. However the site of entry/exit from the central nervous system may be compromised. For the sake of completion they are listed below.

I	Olfactory	Smell
II	Optic	Sight
III	Oculomotor	Movement of eyeball, pupillary accommodation
IV	Trochlear	Movement of eyeball
V	Trigeminal	Sensation and motor control in face, scalp, cornea, nose and mouth
VI	Abducens	Movement of eyeball
VII	Facial	Taste, salivation, tears and facial movement
VIII	Vestibulocochlear	Hearing, position and movement of head
IX	Glossopharyngeal	Taste, swallowing, salivation. Sensation in ear and mouth
X	Vagus	Sensation in ear, pharynx, larynx, oesophagus, viscera. Motor function related to speech, swallowing, cardiovascular system, respiration and gastrointestinal tracts
XI	Accessory motor	Movement of head and shoulder
XII	Hypoglossal	Tongue movement

Symptom management

People with MS can experience a wide range of different symptoms. A survey of 656 people with MS (Kraft, 1986) listed over 14 different symptoms, each experienced by at least 23% of people.

Whatever symptoms someone with MS experiences, they have an impact on a number of different levels and are often all-pervasive, affecting an individual's self-esteem, confidence, role within the family, social life, community involvement and sexuality.

Using a holistic model of care, the types of symptoms experienced can be subdivided into primary, secondary and tertiary. Primary symptoms occur as a direct result of demyelination within the central nervous system, e.g. weakness, bladder dysfunction etc. Secondary symptoms occur as a result of complications caused by a combination of the primary symptoms and insufficient management of the symptom e.g. recurrent urine infections caused by untreated bladder dysfunction. Tertiary symptoms are described as the psychosocial consequences of primary and secondary symptoms, e.g. unemployment, role changes, loss of independence and self-esteem etc. (Holland and Halper, 1999).

Due to the way each symptom impacts on an individual and their family in so many ways a holistic, interdisciplinary team approach to caring for people with MS is imperative. Each of the symptoms which may be experienced in mild-moderate MS are discussed below using this approach; elimination, sexuality, cognitive problems and complications of moderate to severe MS are discussed in subsequent chapters.

Fatigue

Many people with or without MS complain of being tired or fatigued. However, fatigue as a symptom of MS is very different to the fatigue that people experience at the end of a day's work. The MS Council for Clinical Practice Guidelines define it as 'A subjective lack of physical and/or mental energy that is perceived by the individual or care-giver to interfere with usual and desired activities' (Fatigue Guidelines Development Panel members, 1998).

The key to the definition is that fatigue interferes with normal activity and is out of all proportion to any activity undertaken. An individual with MS who is suffering from fatigue may be unable to perform even routine tasks:

> I am exhausted all the time, I can't even prepare the evening meal any more. I slice a few beans or hull some strawberries and then I'm shattered and can't do anything else for an hour or so until I'm rested.
>
> (MJ – wife and mother of two talking about the limitations imposed on her by fatigue)

I break out into a sweat just crossing the room, things I've always taken for granted become such hard work.

(BB – husband and father describing the fatigue experienced during a relapse)

Pathophysiology of fatigue

The pathological mechanisms of fatigue are not well understood and are likely to be multidimensional in nature. As yet no correlation with severity of fatigue and severity of MS has been found, either in terms of disability or with respect to the lesion burden evident on MRI scan.

It is known that fatigue may be either central or peripheral in nature. Central fatigue is caused by transmission of impulses to the muscles fading and becoming unsustainable, whereas peripheral fatigue results from incapacity within the muscle to generate sustained force required to complete the task in hand.

MS fatigue probably results from a combination of both peripheral and central fatigue. Central fatigue is most likely to be caused by lesions in the pyramidal tract, motor cortex or the afferent pathways within the spinal cord. Peripheral fatigue may be due to inherent weakness in the muscle due to lack of appropriate stimuli (Young, 2000).

It is known that MS fatigue has different characteristics to the fatigue experienced after sustained activity by healthy individuals, i.e.

- it comes on easily;
- it prevents physical functioning;
- it is worsened by heat;
- it interferes with responsibilities;
- it causes frequent problems (Krupp *et al.*, 1988).

Role of the nurse

Assessing the person with fatigue

Fatigue can impact on every aspect of a person's life and there may be many factors that exacerbate it, above and beyond demyelination. A thorough assessment of the person with fatigue is therefore essential to allow the secondary and tertiary symptoms resulting from fatigue to be identified and managed as well as tackling any exacerbating factors (see Table 5.1).

Table 5.1 Assessment of the person with fatigue

Assess	Rationale for assessment	Action
Sleeping pattern	Disturbed sleep will exacerbate fatigue	Determine cause of poor sleep and liaise with appropriate interdisciplinary team member
Temperature and pulse	If infection present fatigue will be worse than usual	If temperature elevated, liaise with doctor and administer any medication as prescribed
Send MSU for culture	People with MS are often vulnerable to urine infections	If positive, liaise with doctor and treat appropriately
Normal activity patterns	Is patient too sedentary or too active, have activity levels changed	Liaise with occupational therapist and physiotherapist and advise patient appropriately
Pattern of fatigue	Are there any exacerbating factors, e.g. hot baths	Check patient's understanding of triggers and advise accordingly
Current medication	Some medications can cause drowsiness	Liaise with doctor if there are any concerns
Fluid balance	Patient may have frequency and/or nocturia which disturbs their sleep and causes many trips to the toilet during the day, increasing energy expenditure	Maintain accurate fluid balance, encourage patient to drink 1-1½L fluid daily. Ensure ready access to toilet when required. Liaise with appropriate member of interdisciplinary team re bladder symptoms/ access to toilet etc.
Mood	Low mood may be caused by fatigue or may be an exacerbating factor	Ensure patient has opportunity to voice concerns. Liaise with appropriate members of interdisciplinary team as necessary
Patient's understanding of fatigue	Patient may not be employing appropriate self-help strategies	Educate patient re cause and management of fatigue, refer to occupational therapist and/or physiotherapy as appropriate
Understanding of patient's family/friends etc.	Others may have unrealistic expectations of the person with MS	Educate appropriate individuals re cause and nature of fatigue
Aids and adaptations used at home/work	Lack of appropriate aids and adaptations may cause unnecessary energy expenditure	Refer to occupational therapist

Factors that can worsen MS fatigue

- Heat
- Infection
- Relapse
- Poor posture
- Poor sleeping pattern
- Anxiety
- Stress
- Depression
- Other medical conditions
- Pain
- Nocturia
- Some medications (e.g. baclofen, tizanidine)

All these factors should be taken into account and asked about when assessing someone with MS. Symptoms in MS should not be viewed in isolation as they all impact on each other. For example, someone with frequency of micturition who has no downstairs toilet may suffer from increased fatigue due to constantly having to go up and down stairs. Treating the frequency and providing a commode or preferably a downstairs toilet can solve this relatively easily. This interrelation of symptoms is something that nurses are particularly well placed and skilled at detecting in their initial assessment. They should then liaise with the interdisciplinary team and advise the patient and their family appropriately as detailed below.

Care of the person with fatigue

Fatigue is often poorly understood by family members, friends and work colleagues. The person with MS may also not fully appreciate that their fatigue is part of the MS. Education as to the nature and exacerbating factors of MS fatigue is vital. This enables people to appreciate fatigue as a symptom and allows them the opportunity for clarification and to discuss any pertinent issues. This can prove an effective management strategy in its own right (Clanet *et al.*, 1994).

When planning the care for a patient, it is important to take account of the level of their fatigue. For example if someone is an inpatient, the interdisciplinary team should liaise closely with each other and the patient to ensure that care giving, therapies, tests and treatments are spread out through the day, thus leaving sufficient time for the patient to rest and receive visitors etc. An individual's level of fatigue can vary dramatically from day to day and even hour to hour, and this should be taken into account when planning their care.

Role of the person with MS

There is much that the person with MS can do to help themselves cope with fatigue and the nurse in their role as educator should ensure that the individual is aware of the different strategies which can be used (see Figure 5.2). It is also useful to back up verbal information given with written information; a number of leaflets dealing with fatigue are available from the MS Society among others.

Role of the occupational therapist

Occupational therapists have a major role to play in the management of fatigue. They can advise people on simple energy conserving techniques appropriate to their needs, having first looked at the individual's daily routine and made a thorough assessment of the problems.

Occupational therapists are also able to supply people with any relevant aids and adaptations to help conserve energy, e.g. an electric can opener, a perching stool, grab handles, raised seating etc.

- Pace self and spread activities over the day and/or week
- Prioritise and delegate appropriate activities
- Sit or use a perching stool whenever possible
- Avoid hot baths and saunas prior to any sort of activity
- Avoid the sun when at its hottest – take steps to keep cool during hot weather
- Use home delivery/Internet/catalogues for shopping whenever practical
- Build quality time for self and family/friends into daily routine
- If an activity is planned that will be tiring (e.g. a party/day out) go but ensure a quiet day following the event
- Obtain a disabled badge to minimise distance walked to and from shops/ work etc.
- Ensure some exercise is built into daily routine
- Use appropriate aids and adaptations
- Ask for help if needed

Figure 5.2 Self-help strategies to manage fatigue.

Role of the physiotherapist

Physiotherapists will assess individuals' mobility etc. and work with them to maintain normal movement as far as possible. The physiotherapist is also able to advise on easier ways of transferring or standing etc. and can give advice tailored to the individual's needs regarding exercise. Gradually improving aerobic activity over time in a structured way has been shown to improve stamina and fitness and reduce feelings of anger and depression (Petejan et al., 1996). The physiotherapist is ideally placed to help individuals develop and maintain a structured exercise programme.

Role of the doctor

The doctor should examine and assess the patient thoroughly. It is important to rule out any underlying medical condition (e.g. anaemia) which may be contributing to the fatigue. The doctor should also review the patient's medication and ensure this is not aggravating the fatigue. Many different medications can cause drowsiness and some of the more common medications used in MS, e.g. anti-spasticity medications or those used in pain relief may fall into this category.

The doctor may also prescribe medication to treat the fatigue itself. However, this should not be done until the interdisciplinary team has made a thorough assessment of potential causes and solutions.

Vitamin B12 injections

Although there have been no trials performed, regular intramuscular injections of vitamin B12 (hydroxocobalamin) appear to relieve symptoms of MS fatigue in some people. It is unclear whether the mode of action is placebo or not. It is usually worth trying the injections at a frequency of one every 4 weeks for a period of 4–6 months; if after this time the individual has not noted any easing of their fatigue then the injections can be discontinued as they are unlikely to prove effective.

Amantadine

The only readily available medication in the UK that has been shown to be effective against fatigue is amantadine. Its mode of action is unknown although various studies have shown it to be effective in treating fatigue in MS (Cohen and Fisher, 1989; Krupp et al., 1995).

Amantadine is generally well tolerated and any side effects are usually mild. Possible side effects include constipation, vivid dreams, nausea, anxiety, insomnia and hyperactivity. Patients should be advised to take 100mg amantadine at breakfast time with the potential to add another 100mg at lunch time should this prove necessary. Amantadine should be taken no later than 2 pm to counteract potential problems with insomnia and vivid dreams. Modafanil is now also available and can be effective in treating fatigue in MS.

Pemoline

Pemoline is a central nervous system stimulant, which can be used to treat MS fatigue. However studies have shown that patients only benefit from pemoline at higher doses which are in turn associated with more side effects (Weinshenker *et al.*, 1992; Krupp *et al.*, 1995). These include anorexia, irritability and insomnia.

It should be remembered that while medications may be necessary and certainly have their place in treating MS fatigue, first line treatment should be support, education and advice from appropriate members of the interdisciplinary team.

Mobility

Problems mobilising are possibly the most well-recognised manifestation of MS and one of the first symptoms that most people think of when they imagine someone with MS. The majority of people with MS will experience some sort of mobility problem during their life. There are four main symptoms, which directly affect an individual's ability to walk in mild-moderate MS, i.e.

- ataxia
- poor balance
- weakness
- spasms

These are discussed in more detail below.

Impact of reduced mobility

Whether an individual is experiencing mild weakness or is unable to mobilise independently, the impact on their lives is great and multi-faceted. Dimensions of self that can be affected (i.e. tertiary symptoms) include self-confidence and esteem, personal security, sexuality, family role, elimination and independence.

> Because I'm unsteady and slur my words people sometimes think I'm drunk.
>
> (SJ – single woman working in a bank)

> I'd only had an orange juice but stumbled coming out of a pub with the family. This guy started a fight because I bumped into him and I've never felt so low. I couldn't even protect myself, never mind the family. It really brought home to me how vulnerable MS has made me.
>
> (MT – husband, father of three and factory worker)

> It's not so much that I can't hold on until I get to the toilet, it's just that it takes me so long to get there that I wet myself.
>
> (LM – husband and retired teacher)

Pathophysiology of factors affecting mobility

Ataxia

Ataxia is a relatively common symptom in MS and is typified by uncoordinated movements of the legs when walking. The upper limbs may also occasionally become ataxic and uncoordinated. The pathology is not clearly defined but is likely to be due to a combination of both demyelination and axonal loss, particularly in the cerebellum, basal ganglia and posterior fossa (Young, 2000).

Balance

The balance centres are located in the cerebellum and are commonly affected by MS plaques. As a result, people with MS often feel unsteady; this can be a particular problem when turning quickly or when in an open space with no source of support (e.g. when crossing a road).

Weakness

Weakness is the result of delayed electrical impulses due to demyelination within the spinal cord or less often the brain. Weakness in MS primarily originates from lesions within the central nervous system rather than problems in the muscles themselves. Thus some repetitive exercises (if performed incorrectly) may only cause worsening fatigue rather than increasing strength within the muscle (Schapiro and Schneider, 1997).

Spasms

Spasticity is an upper motor neurone symptom and results from involvement of the para-pyramidal tracts. These tracts control the interneuronal networks in the spinal cord so influencing the lower motor neurones. When the balance between inhibition and excitation of the neurones is disrupted so that the excitatory stimuli are strongest then spasticity can result (Barnes, 2000a). This in turn may cause increased tone and resistance to movement to develop.

A spasm is a sudden involuntary muscle contraction, which can vary greatly in severity. Spasms tend to be at their worst when an individual is relaxing, e.g. in bed at night. Spasms may also be triggered by handling the affected limb and can be caused or sometimes relieved by altering the position of the limb. Severe spasticity and spasms and potential complications which may arise from these will be discussed in Chapter 11.

NB Treatment of spasticity should only be undertaken when it is causing problems. People with MS often require a degree of spasticity to provide support for otherwise weak limbs so allowing them to walk around.

Role of the nurse

While treating mobility problems is primarily the domain of the physiotherapist and occupational therapist, the nurse is ideally placed to assess the impact of reduced mobility on all other aspects of the patient's life. The nurse must ensure that they understand the management and treatment options available and that they discuss these with the person with MS. By providing the individual with support and information the patient is then in a position to make an informed choice about treatment options (Melia, 1998).

The nurse may also be one of the first members of the interdisciplinary team to detect that someone is having difficulties with their mobility and is then responsible for liaising with the GP/neurologist, physiotherapist and occupational therapist etc.

Role of the physiotherapist

Once a patient is referred to the physiotherapist, a full assessment will be made to determine the extent and nature of the problem. The physiotherapist may then see the patient regularly over a period of time, working with them to maximise their potential. The physiotherapist may also prescribe a personalised exercise programme for the patient to follow at home.

The physiotherapist is usually responsible for providing any walking aids which may be required, e.g. sticks, elbow crutches, strollers, wheel-chairs etc. Orthotic devices may also be helpful and referral to an ortho-tist may be required.

All newly diagnosed people with MS should ideally be seen by a phys-iotherapist as should anyone who is new to the service locally and has not seen a physiotherapist recently (Freeman *et al.*, 1997). Patients often develop compensatory strategies when coping with a weakness or ataxia such as favouring their stronger side or developing postural changes. Overtime these compensations can lead to musculoskeletal complications and the physiotherapist is ideally placed to correct these 'bad habits' and encourage the individual to use normal movement as far as possible.

Walking aids

These come in many shapes and sizes. Walking aids should be viewed as tools to enable people with MS to get to places they may not otherwise be able to access. Many people feel they are 'giving in' when they start to use a stick or wheelchair. However, in the same way that a second handrail may allow someone to be independent going up and down stairs, so a walking aid can allow someone to be independently mobile.

A stick may also give someone more confidence in other ways. Not only does it increase their mobility and stability, it also lets other people know that they may need more time and space to get anywhere. It also stops strangers jumping to the conclusion that the individual is drunk; this is something many people with MS have experienced at some time and is understandably very distressing.

It is the role of the nurse to help people who have been given a walking aid for the first time come to terms with its use. People should be encour-aged to view it as a move towards increasing independence and a way to get to places with friends and family that would otherwise be difficult to access.

Role of the orthotist

Some patients require an orthosis of some description (e.g. an AFO – ankle foot orthosis). The most common cause for needing an orthosis is when someone has foot drop, i.e. they have a weak ankle and as a result are unable to lead with their heel in the normal way when taking a step. This in turn makes them vulnerable to tripping and potentially falling for no obvious reason. Individuals with foot drop also often find that the top of their shoe becomes very scuffed on their affected side. An ankle foot orthosis is worn inside the shoe and allows them to walk in a more normal way.

The proper use of AFOs may also help to reduce spasticity and maintain correct positioning of the affected foot and ankle. They may also have secondary benefits in reducing fatigue, increasing stability and reducing the likelihood of trips and falls.

Role of the occupational therapist

The occupational therapist often works closely with the physiotherapist in this context. They can give advice on wheelchairs and any specialised seating that may be required.

The occupational therapist will also assess and advise the individual on any aids and adaptations that may improve their function around the house or workplace. For example, a perching stool to provide support for people who cannot stand for long; or a trolley to allow them to carry drinks and food etc. from one room to another. The occupational therapists are also able to advise patients on the management of their fatigue, which can impact on their mobility and vice versa.

Role of the doctor

The doctor may be the first member of the interdisciplinary team to detect a problem and should then refer the patient to the appropriate interdisciplinary team member (usually the physiotherapist in the first instance). The doctor is also responsible for prescribing any appropriate medication.

There is no one medication that can make someone walk better. However certain medications targeted at specific problems (i.e. spasticity) may help some people.

Lioresal (baclofen)

This is the medication that is most commonly used to treat stiffness and spasms. It acts on the central nervous system to relieve increased tone and can be given in either tablet or liquid form. The dose for each individual must be titrated carefully as it is difficult to predict the therapeutic dose for any given individual prior to starting treatment. Some people will gain relief at a dose of 5mg whereas others may require 40mg three times a day to achieve the desired effect.

Baclofen should always be increased and decreased slowly. The usual starting dose is 5–10mg and the amount can be increased every few days by similar amounts until symptoms improve. If someone is taking more than 30mg daily they should not stop the baclofen suddenly but should reduce the dose by 5–10mg every few days. If high doses of baclofen are stopped suddenly it can cause hallucinations, an increase in spasms and restlessness.

Baclofen is usually well tolerated and any initial problems often settle down. The most common difficulty can be that as the increased tone is reduced the limbs become much weaker and for some individuals this may significantly affect their mobility. This effect can be seen at any dose of baclofen depending on how sensitive the individual is. Once the dose is reduced or the baclofen stopped the effect is reversed. Other potential side effects include drowsiness, dizziness and difficulty sleeping.

Tizanidine (Zanaflex)

This works in a similar way to baclofen although it has less potential to cause limb weakness. The usual starting dose is 2–4mg and the dose is increased and reduced as necessary in the same way as baclofen. The recommended therapeutic dose is between 24–36mg daily (UK Tizanidine Trial Group, 1994) although some people achieve relief at lower doses.

It is recommended that patients who are on baclofen and/or tizanidine have three monthly blood tests. Both medications have the ability to affect liver function and by checking the liver enzymes in a routine blood test any problems can be detected before there is any damage caused.

Other drugs, which are less commonly used, include dantrolene and diazepam. Dantrolene works directly on the muscles and is also potentially hepatotoxic. Diazepam is rarely used as a long-term treatment for spasticity now but may very occasionally be useful at night due to its sedative effects.

Pain

In the past MS was regarded as a painless disease. However it is now well recognised that pain is experienced by over half of all people with MS and can be one of the worst symptoms experienced for approximately 20% people (MS Society, 1997).

Pain experienced by people with MS may be caused in a number of different ways. Demyelination of axons may result in misinterpretation of nerve transmissions, resulting in the perception of pain in a particular part of the body. People with MS are also prone to musculoskeletal pain due to problems with fatigue and weakness. It is important to distinguish between the two types, as the recommended treatments are very different.

Someone with musculoskeletal pain will often benefit from painkillers such as paracetamol or brufen. Pain caused directly by demyelination cannot be treated effectively by the usual analgesics, as these are unable to cross the blood–brain barrier and affect the central nervous system, which is the origin of the problem.

Pain is very subjective and is best understood and described by the person experiencing it. Nurses are well equipped to detect and assess pain and its effects on an individual. Pain can impact on all aspects of life and likewise factors such as mood, support network, religion and culture will have an impact on an individual's response to pain. All these factors should be taken into account when caring for someone in pain.

Classification of pain in MS

MS pain can take many forms and a classification system has been devised (Moulin *et al.*, 1988).

Acute pain

This is usually experienced as intermittent episodes with a sudden and spontaneous onset. People tend to describe this type of pain variously as intense, sharp, shooting or burning.

Acute pain includes problems such as trigeminal neuralgia, headaches, limb pain etc. It can signify an underlying inflammatory process so any new onset of acute pain should be properly investigated.

Sub-acute pain

This results from an acute worsening of symptoms either during relapse or as a result of complications of MS, e.g. optic neuritis, pressure sores, urine infections etc.

Chronic pain

This is defined as any pain which lasts longer than a month, e.g. dysasthesia (i.e. an uncomfortable and abnormal sensation), back pain, banding (a tight feeling around the chest) and spasms.

It should be noted that people with MS are just as likely to experience pain unrelated to MS as any one else is and the cause of their pain should always be investigated with an open mind.

Types of pain

Acute pain

Trigeminal neuralgia

This can occur in people with or without MS although someone with MS is 400 times more likely to experience trigeminal neuralgia then someone without MS. In MS it is caused by demyelination of the trigeminal nerve near the point of entry at the pons (Maloni, 2000).

The pain can be excruciating and can be triggered by chewing, smiling, talking, temperature change, eating and drinking, even a light breeze may cause an attack.

Headache

The link between headache and MS is unclear although it is known that people with MS have a greater frequency of headache than the general population. They may be caused as a result of the inflammatory process or may be due to the increased stress of living with MS.

Optic neuritis

The optic nerve may become swollen due to the inflammatory process inherent in MS. This may, in turn, put a strain on the surrounding meninges causing pain. The pain is usually stabbing or nagging in nature.

Chronic pain

Dysasthesia

Dysasthesia is defined as an uncomfortable abnormal sensation and is very common in MS. It usually affects the extremities but may be experienced in any part of the body. This type of sensation often provokes particularly vivid descriptions by patients.

Patient descriptions

- 'I feel as though I've got boiling tea inside my legs.'
- 'It feels as though I'm wearing tight pants made of rotting leather.'
- 'I feel like I've got ants crawling under my skin.'

Common words used by patients to describe their dysasthesia are:

- burning
- itching
- pins and needles
- crawling
- heavy
- pressing
- tight
- prickling
- tingling
- dull
- nagging
- numb

Many people also describe the feeling of having a tight band around their chest (known, unsurprisingly, as banding). Others will experience a feeling in their hands and feet as though they are constantly wearing gloves or boots.

Dysasthetic pain is caused by lesions in the dorsal column of the spinal cord (Maloni, 2000). The axons in the dorsal column transmit impulses concerned with movement, joint position sense and discriminative touch (Crossman and Neary, 1998).

Musculoskeletal pain

People with MS are more vulnerable to aches and sprains, trips and strains than others. To compensate for weakness in one or more areas of the body, individuals often unconsciously develop 'bad habits' to allow them to function. This can in turn put a strain on muscles and joints in the stronger part of their body so potentially leading to musculoskeletal pain. Physiotherapy is essential in resolving this type of pain.

Spasms

Spasms can be very painful and are characterised by flexor and/or extensor cramping of the muscles. They are usually felt in the legs and may be exacerbated by infection, constipation, a full bladder, touch, position or change in temperature.

Pain management

Role of the nurse

It can be seen from the above descriptions that an accurate assessment of the pain is necessary to determine the most appropriate management. The nurse is skilled in determining the type, degree and impact of any pain experienced.

It should always be remembered that everyone has a different pain threshold and that pain is very much a subjective experience. The nurse will need all her skills of observation, open questioning and empathy to make a full assessment. Many factors outside the physical realm will have an impact on the individual's perception of pain and the coping strategies they employ. Social and family support, culture, religion, age, gender and responsibilities will all affect the way someone copes with and responds to pain (McFarland and McFarlane, 1997). Fear, anxiety, anger and grief, which are all a natural response to the unpredictable nature of MS and to pain itself, will also aggravate the pain and will themselves be heightened by it. It is the role of the interdisciplinary team to try and break this spiral of pain and fear.

When making their assessment the nurse should focus both on the pain itself and on its wider impact (see Figure 5.3). During time spent with and near the patient, the nurse should observe their non-verbal cues – are they restless and finding it difficult to get comfortable? do they seem

---

- Where is the pain?
- Can the patient point to the area?
- Can the patient describe the pain?
- Is it constant or fluctuating?
- Is there anything that makes it worse or that provides relief?
- How long have they had the pain?
- What medication are they taking?
- Is their medication effective?
- What else have they tried?
- Do they use any complementary therapies?
- Are they effective?
- Do they employ any other coping strategies?
- Has their appetite been affected?
- Are they sleeping well?
- Are their bladder and bowels functioning normally?
- Is there any sign of infection?

Figure 5.3 Assessing the person with pain in MS.

depressed and/or withdrawn? do they have good family/social support? what do their facial expressions convey? are they able to relax?

The nurse should also record the patient's vital signs and the use of a pain scale such as a visual analogue scale is highly recommended. This can take the form of a line of standard length with each end representing the extremes of 'the worst pain ever felt' and 'no pain', the patient marks a vertical line at whichever point they feel approximates best to the degree of pain they are experiencing. This not only provides a measure of the patient's pain but may also be used to assess the effectiveness of any interventions employed.

Having built up a picture of the patient's pain and their coping strategies, it is imperative that the information is shared fully with the interdisciplinary team and the patient to ensure a holistic approach to the management of their pain.

Throughout the nurse's involvement with the patient he/she should be constantly reassessing the patient's level of pain and the effectiveness of any interventions employed.

The nurse should also be involved in helping the patient to develop appropriate coping strategies. Pain may be eased by simple interventions such as changing position and supporting the affected area. Applying heat or cold to the area may also provide some relief (although care must be taken if the individual has reduced sensation and is unable to tell if something is too hot or cold). Relaxation techniques are beneficial generally for the person with MS but can be particularly helpful in managing pain. These can be something as simple as a breathing exercise or listening to a relaxation tape. The nurse can find some quiet time to spend with the patient to talk them through these different options and find something that will suit them. Alternatively the patient can be referred to the MS specialist nurse for further support.

Other techniques that can be useful include massage, stress management, exercise programmes, visualisation and distraction. (Distraction is simply an activity that distracts the patient from their pain, e.g. going out somewhere, meeting friends and family, listening to music etc.) The MS specialist nurse can also advise patients about these different techniques.

Role of the doctor

The doctor will make a thorough assessment of the patient and their pain. It is important that any cause other than MS is ruled out. The doctor should work closely with other members of the interdisciplinary team and the patient throughout.

One of the doctor's main roles apart from diagnosing the cause of the pain is in prescribing medication to relieve the pain. The more readily available analgesics such as paracetamol may be useful in relieving musculoskeletal pain but will not affect pain resulting directly from lesions in the central nervous system. This type of pain requires medication that can cross the blood–brain barrier and often anti-epileptics or anti-depressants are useful in this context. Some of the more commonly used medications are listed below.

Amitriptyline

Recommended for dysasthetic pain. Recommended starting dose 10–25mg increasing to 50–75mg with a maximum dose of 100–150mg as required. Amitriptyline is usually taken at night as it can cause drowsiness. Other potential side effects include a dry mouth, blurred vision, urinary retention and constipation.

Imipramine

This is very similar to amitriptyline and should be used in the same way; it tends to be less sedating.

Carbamazepine (Tegretol)

Indicated for trigeminal neuralgia and dysasthesia. The usual starting dose is 100–200mg daily, which can be increased gradually to a maximum of 1.6g until a satisfactory effect is found. Most people take a dose of 200–600mg to relieve MS pain. Potential side effects include nausea, dizziness, sedation, weakness, hepatotoxicity and constipation. Patients should also be counselled regarding contraception as carbamazepine could negate the action of certain types of contraceptive pill.

Gabapentin (Neurontin)

Indicated for trigeminal neuralgia and dysasthesia. Recommended starting dose of 300mg daily building gradually to 900mg and then increased according to best response up to a maximum of 1.2g. Gabapentin should be stopped gradually if necessary. Potential side effects include sedation, dizziness, fatigue, nystagmus and occasionally increased weakness (information taken from British National Formulary, 1999).

Cannabis

A significant minority of people with MS use cannabis to relieve symptoms of pain and spasticity. At present this remains illegal and patients can be and are prosecuted for possessing cannabis. Patients also run the risk of not knowing exactly what they are buying, whether it has been mixed with anything or the plants sprayed with anything; the purity of the cannabis may also vary unbeknown to the patient. Despite this many people continue to use it and the anecdotal evidence shows that cannabis can be very effective in relieving these symptoms.

Most people prefer not to smoke it but either make a tea with it, bake it in a cake or biscuits or mix it in yoghurt etc. When taking the cannabis orally, patients must be careful to allow time for the cannabis to be absorbed properly before deciding that it isn't working and taking more; it is very easy to take too much in this way which can result in hallucinations and paranoia.

There is currently a nationwide trial of cannabis underway (known as the CAMS trial – cannabis in MS). It is hoped that the trial will demonstrate the effectiveness of cannabis in relieving symptoms of spasticity in particular. The trial will also allow doctors to determine the most effective dose for patients and to observe for any possible side effects. If the trial is successful it is hoped that cannabis will be available on prescription for people with MS in the next few years.

Some pain caused by MS is extremely difficult to treat and in these circumstances referral to a specialised pain management team should be considered.

Role of the physiotherapist

The physiotherapist can advise the patient with respect to exercise and position. They will assess the patient's gait etc. and advise the patient on the best way to move around minimising any strain on the painful area.

Physiotherapists may also be able to use electrical treatment, acupuncture, massage or heat treatments to relieve certain types of pain. TENs machines may also be helpful in a few cases and the physiotherapist can advise the patient on their use.

Role of the occupational therapist

The occupational therapist is able to assess seating needs and provide any aids or adaptations that may be required. This can be particularly relevant where pain is aggravated by positional factors.

Role of the psychologist

A few patients may benefit from referral to a psychologist who can help them develop more appropriate coping strategies.

Visual disturbances

The visual system comprises the eyes, the optic tract and the visual cortex in the occipital lobe. In order to see and interpret what is being seen, all these separate components of the visual system, and the tracts between them, must be functioning correctly.

Most people with MS will experience some visual disturbances at some stage. This is often one of the presenting signs of MS.

Optic neuritis

This is the most common visual problem experienced by people with MS and is caused by inflammation and demyelination of the optic nerve. It is characterised by visual loss in one eye with associated pain behind the eye. This usually improves over a few weeks and responds well to steroid treatment (Beck *et al.*, 1992). The patient usually experiences haziness or blurring of vision and may notice some loss of colour vision. People may sometimes experience flashes of light in the affected eye or may find bright lights uncomfortable.

Recovery from an attack of optic neuritis is usually good, however repeated attacks may lead to some permanent loss of vision and the individual may then require visual aids.

Abnormal visual fields

The visual field describes the range of vision, both central and peripheral that the patient has. Any defects in the field of vision (i.e. field defects) are experienced as blind spots or 'holes' by the individual.

Double vision

A weakening in the co-ordination and strength of the eye muscles may cause double vision. Again this often resolves spontaneously over time and usually responds well to steroids if required. Patients may find it helpful to cover one eye with a patch when reading, watching TV etc. as this can minimise the double vision. Care should be taken to cover both eyes in turn so that one particular eye is not left strained.

Nystagmus

If present this can be elicited by asking the patient to follow your finger to their extreme of vision either from side to side or up and down. If nystagmus is present the eye(s) will appear to jump at one or other of the extremes. The patient experiences this as a flickering or jumping of their vision which can be quite disconcerting. This symptom often settles on its own.

Speech

The most common form of speech problem experienced by people with MS is dysarthria, i.e. incoordination of the muscles of the lips, tongue and face which are necessary to form speech. It is typified by a slurring and/or slowing of speech and people are often very self conscious about the problem.

Slurred speech is often found in association with ataxia.

It is unclear exactly where the lesion(s) which causes dysarthria are sited but it is thought to be most likely in the region of the brainstem (Clanet *et al.*, 1994).

The nurse should ensure that the patient understands the problem is part of the MS and as with many MS symptoms the problem will be worse when the patient is tired, stressed, hot or has an infection. It is also important that the patient feels able to explain the nature of the problem to their family, friends and colleagues. The nurse may well be able to facilitate this. Referral to a speech and language therapist may also be required and can be very helpful.

Swallowing

The muscles in the throat that facilitate swallowing may become weak and uncoordinated. One of the first signs is that the individual tends to cough and splutter when drinking. An assessment by the speech and language therapist is vital and they will advise the patient and their family about the importance of maintaining a correct posture and head position when swallowing. Swallowing problems tend to occur more commonly in people with moderate–severe MS and will be discussed in more detail in Chapter 11.

Temperature control

People with MS often find that they feel hot when the rest of the family feel cold or vice versa.

I'll be stood with the front door wide open and only a T-shirt on in the middle of winter and still be hot, while my husband is sat next to the fire with two jumpers on.

(MC – housewife)

There is little that can be done to resolve this symptom other than advising all concerned that it is part of the MS and perhaps urging some measure of compromise. It should be remembered that the person with MS does not feel hot to the touch and it is more a problem of perception than actual temperature change. Care should be taken to differentiate between menopausal symptoms and changes in temperature perception due to MS in women.

Cold feet

This is a common symptom in MS and is often a problem for both the person with MS and their partner who shares a bed with them. The feet may be cold to the touch or may feel normal but be perceived as feeling cold by the person with MS. This is a result of lesions in the centre of the brain, which are responsible for temperature perception. If the feet are cold to the touch it may be due to the nerves controlling the diameter of the surface capillaries which are affected. MS does not affect the circulatory system as such. Keeping the feet warm with socks or an electric blanket etc. may be sufficient to manage the problem. Cold feet often warm up temporarily when the individual has steroids, although the administration of steroids purely because someone has cold feet is not advised.

Swollen ankles

Swollen ankles often occur in association with reduced mobility. They are caused by pooling of the lymphatic fluid due to reduced activity of the calf muscles. Diuretics are rarely helpful and are more likely to exacerbate any urinary problems for the person with MS. The most effective treatment is to increase activity as much as possible and when resting to elevate the feet so that they are higher than the hips. Correctly fitted support stockings may also be helpful.

The swelling is often greater in summer due to the increasing dilation of the lymph channels in the heat. Swollen ankles often adversely affect an individual's body image and can make relatively simple tasks such as finding a pair of shoes to fit, particularly difficult.

If the swelling is associated with dyspnoea, coughing and generally feeling unwell, the patient should be advised to see the doctor as soon as possible as it may indicate some cardiac involvement separate to the problems caused by MS.

Management of relapse

A relapse is defined as the recurrence of old symptoms or the appearance of new symptoms lasting for 48 hours or more.

Traditionally acute relapses are treated with steroids. It is also important to manage any symptoms resulting from the relapse appropriately and to ensure that the patient gets sufficient rest balanced with appropriate exercise.

Steroids have been shown to be effective in shortening the time taken to recover from relapses. However they do not have any effect in the longer term either on the extent of recovery from the relapse or on prognosis (Barnes, 2000b).

The mode of action of steroids is not fully understood. However it is known that they act to suppress the immune system which is known to have a central role in the onset of relapses (Pitzalis *et al.*, 1997). Steroids are also known to stabilise the blood–brain barrier, which is damaged during lesion formation. Gadolinium enhanced MRI scans taken within hours of a dose of steroids show almost complete absence of lesion enhancement. This effect is lost very soon after stopping steroids, indicating that other mechanisms must also be involved (Barnes, 2000b).

Oral versus intravenous steroids

A survey of UK neurologists regarding their use of steroids in MS, showed that there is little consensus in terms of the use of oral versus intravenous steroids when treating relapse. Indeed there was little consensus shown in terms of the optimum dosing regime to be used (Tremlett *et al.*, 1998). Studies have shown that there is no significant benefit to using either oral or intravenous steroids in terms of outcomes such as a reduction in disability measured by the Expanded Disability Status Scale (EDSS) (Barnes *et al.*, 1997).

However, there are likely to be significant cost savings in using oral steroids rather than intravenous steroids (Tremlett and Wiles, 1999).

The benefits of using oral steroids rather than intravenous go beyond that of cost savings; they can be taken at home with minimal disruption to the patient's life. Having said this, however, some patients do still require admission to hospital for intravenous steroids due to the severity of their relapse. The benefits of admission for the patient are that the appropriate members of the interdisciplinary team can see them during their stay and appropriate symptom management can be commenced. The patient may also benefit from the enforced rest experienced during a hospital stay.

Care of the patient taking steroids

Oral steroids

If patients are prescribed oral steroids they are more likely to liaise solely with their GP and/or neurologist and MS specialist nurse.

The recommended regime is either:

- Oral prednisolone on a reducing dose from 60mg over 3 weeks, or preferably
- Oral methylprednisolone 500mg daily for 5 days

The latter has been shown to be the more effective regime of the two (Sellebjerg *et al.*, 1998).

Patients should be advised to take their medication with food as oral steroids can cause dyspepsia or ulceration of the stomach wall. Wherever possible the steroids should be enteric coated or a suitable antacid should be prescribed to be taken at the same time.

Patients should be advised of any potential side effects such as difficulty sleeping and facial flushing. However these tend to be minimal. Ideally patients should have a contact number such as that of the MS specialist nurse should they need any further advice. The MS specialist nurse or GP should also monitor the effectiveness of the steroids and liaise with the neurologist as necessary.

Intravenous methylprednisolone

The most common regime prescribed is 1g daily for 3 days or alternatively 0.5g daily for 5 days (Barnes, 2000a).

Patients may be admitted to a day ward for administration of intravenous methylprednisolone (IVMP) which often provides an acceptable compromise between prescribing oral steroids or admitting patients to a bed on the neurology ward.

When a patient is admitted, a full assessment of their needs should be made by the nursing staff and referrals to appropriate members of the interdisciplinary team made.

Intravenous steroids tend to be well tolerated, the more common side effects and appropriate actions are as follows:

- metallic taste in mouth – slow down infusion rate;
- pain and redness around venflon site – resite venflon and observe patient for signs of infection;
- glycosuria – check urine daily for glucose, if present advise patients to reduce sugar intake for a few days;
- insomnia/increased activity – ensure infusion given in the morning, encourage the patient to rest even if unable to sleep; advise patient not to overdo it;
- facial flushing – should settle once the steroids are completed;
- menstrual irregularities – should settle quite quickly;
- euphoria – if steroid induced should settle quickly once steroids completed.

Patients are often concerned about the potential for weight gain when given steroids. There is no evidence that this is a recognised complication in patients given steroids over short periods as recommended above.

There are no benefits for people with MS in taking long-term steroids; indeed this is much more likely to lead to complications. There is also no fixed frequency that an individual can have steroids in any 12-month period. Most neurologists will try to limit the number of steroid courses an individual receives due to concerns over the cumulative side effects of steroids over time.

Fears of osteoporosis developing in people with MS due to the effects of repeated steroid treatment appear to be largely unfounded. It is felt to be more likely that the recognised reduction in bone density in MS is due to low levels of mobility in patients rather than to steroids (Schwid et al., 1996).

CHAPTER 6

Bladder and bowel symptoms in MS

Introduction

The majority of patients with MS will experience some problems with bladder and bowel function at some stage during the course of their disease. The exact figures are unknown, but likely to be in excess of 80% (Namey, 1997).

In a recent survey of patients with MS by the MS Society (MS Society, 1997), 66% of people admitted to experiencing bladder and bowel symptoms at the time of the survey. The impact of bladder and/or bowel dysfunction on every aspect of life can be huge, and yet these symptoms are among those most readily treated.

This chapter will examine the normal anatomy and physiology of elimination and how this can be affected in MS. Treatments, therapies and management of symptoms are also discussed. The nurse's role in managing elimination problems is central.

Anatomy and physiology of bladder function

The bladder is a collapsible, muscular, bag-like structure. Its function is to store and expel urine via the urethra. Control of the bladder is exerted via the frontal lobes, brainstem and spinal cord. All of these centres can be directly affected by demyelination.

Frontal lobes in cortex   These exert voluntary control over voiding by sending appropriate impulses to the pontine micturition centre (PMC)

Pontine micturition centre is in the pons	This exerts a more subtle control of bladder function via a network of neurones from other sub-cortical regions Information is received from the detrusor muscle via the sacral micturition centre in the spinal cord and is interpreted within the pontine micturition centre
Sacral micturition centre S2, 3 and 4	This links with the pontine micturition centre – the parasympathetic nerves link with the detrusor muscle (so causing contractions) there is also a link with the internal sphincter causing relaxation of the external urethral sphincter which is controlled via the pudendal nerve (allowing voluntary control of this sphincter) so allowing voiding to occur
Sympathetic nerves T 9 – 12	These cause relaxation of the detrusor muscle and contraction of the internal sphincter, so preventing voiding

In summary the bladder walls consist of the detrusor muscle which contracts under the influence of the parasympathetic nerves controlled via the sacral micturition centre (SMC), and relax under influence of sympathetic nerves controlled via T9–12 in the spinal cord. At the base of the bladder wall is the internal sphincter which is also controlled by sympathetic and parasympathetic fibres. Sympathetic fibres cause contraction of this sphincter, and parasympathetic fibres cause it to relax. The external sphincter is under voluntary control via the pudendal nerve and ultimately the frontal lobes, which initiate and inhibit micturition depending on the appropriateness of voiding at any particular time.

The average bladder capacity is 300–500mls. Most people feel the urge to void when the bladder contains approximately 200mls of urine, however bladder contractions are normally inhibited until it is socially acceptable to pass urine. Most people urinate 4–6 times in 24 hours and produce on average 1ml of urine every minute.

Common urinary symptoms in MS

Frequency	The need to pass urine more frequently than every 2–3 hours. 'I just get settled when I have to get up and go to the toilet again, sometimes it can be every 20 minutes and I can't get anything done' (BJ – mother of two)
Nocturia	The need to get up more than once nightly to void. 'It's so disheartening, I'm so tired but keep waking up to go to the toilet, it takes me ages to get off again leaving me even more tired the day after' (ST – warehouse foreman and father of two)
Urgency	A strong desire to void that cannot be postponed until it is socially acceptable to do so.

	'Once I feel the need to go, I have to go straight away, no matter what I'm doing. I had to go in the middle of a meeting last week – it was that or wet myself' (AM – part-time lecturer)
Hesitancy	A difficulty initiating voiding. 'Sometimes I sit there for 20 minutes and nothing happens and then it happens and I'm OK again for a couple of hours' (BC – father of two)
Incontinence	A loss of control of voiding which may present as leaking, dribbling or loss of larger amounts of urine. 'I was stood in the queue at the supermarket and it just came away from me with no warning, I didn't know where to put myself' (LM – housewife)
Incomplete emptying	The bladder fails to empty fully and the individual may retain a sensation of urine remaining in the bladder. This is often related to frequency and urgency and may cause recurrent urine infections
Urinary tract infection	This is more common in people with MS and may cause burning or pain on micturition. Symptoms include cloudy, offensive smelling urine, and general malaise. Urinary tract infections may also cause an exacerbation of MS

The symptoms reported by a patient give an indication of the cause, but often further investigations are necessary to determine fully the nature of the problem and hence the appropriate treatment recommended.

Causes of urinary symptoms

Detrusor hyper-reflexia

The detrusor muscle (i.e. the bladder wall) experiences spontaneous waves of contraction. This results in symptoms of urgency and frequency and often leads to incomplete bladder emptying. It is thought to be caused by a block in the connection between the parasympathetic and the sympathetic nerves due to spinal cord plaques. In effect the bladder (or detrusor muscle) behaves in the same way as reflexes elsewhere in the body that can become very brisk and which react by contracting strongly when tapped by a tendon hammer. That is the bladder contracts without warning and often incompletely so people experience urgency, frequency and sometimes incontinence as a result.

Detrusor – sphincter dysynergy

Normal bladder function is dependent on the detrusor muscle contracting as the external sphincter relaxes. However, if the bladder is isolated by plaques from the frontal lobes (which control the external sphincter) and the parasympathetic fibres, then the detrusor contracts while at the same time, the external sphincter remains closed. This often leads to incomplete emptying and hesitancy.

Detrusor areflexia

The detrusor muscle does not contract efficiently, leading to incomplete emptying, i.e. the bladder does not empty fully due to incomplete transmission of the nervous impulses in the spinal cord.

As with many symptoms experienced by people with MS, bladder problems impact on and are affected by many factors. Many people find their lives centred around the toilet and any outing, even to the local shops, has to be planned depending on where the accessible toilets are situated. Table 6.1 lists the symptoms of MS that can make elimination more difficult. It also lists factors unrelated to MS that can aggravate elimination problems such as a high intake of caffeine, alcohol and/or carbonated drinks, all of which can irritate the bladder and act as mild diuretics so causing frequency and urgency.

Table 6.2 lists the different aspects of self that bladder dysfunction can affect. It can be seen that these are many and far-reaching. As was discussed in Chapter 5, every symptom experienced in MS impacts on other symptoms and aspects of self. It often falls to the nurse to try and unravel these symptoms and a thorough assessment is key to this process.

Table 6.1 Factors which can exacerbate bladder symptoms

- Relapse
- Urinary tract infection
- Reduced mobility
- Spasticity
- Spasms
- Constipation
- Accessibility of toilet
- Reduced peri-anal sensation
- Moderate to high caffeine intake
- Smoking
- Fizzy drinks
- Menstruation
- Difficulty in removing clothing prior to voiding
- Multiple births - weak pelvic floor

Table 6.2 Aspects of self that can be affected by bladder dysfunction

* Self-confidence
* Sexuality
* Body image
* Skin integrity
* Bowel function
* Sleep
* Mood
* Ability to leave house
* Relationships
* Fatigue

Assessing bladder symptoms in people with MS

The nurse is central in the assessment and management of bladder problems. A complete nursing assessment of the symptoms and their impact is the key to establishing an accurate diagnosis of the cause of the problems and determining the most appropriate management.

1. How often do you go to the toilet?
2. Is your toilet upstairs or downstairs?
3. How good is your mobility?
4. How often are you up overnight to pass urine?
5. Do you get back to sleep again quickly?
6. Does your partner need to get up with you?
7. Do you feel that you empty your bladder fully when you go?
8. Do you find it hard to start passing urine, even though you feel the need to go?
9. When you feel that you need to pass urine do you have to go straight away?
10. Do you ever find that you cannot get to the toilet in time and have an 'accident'?
11. Do you need to wear pads?
12. How much and what are you drinking?
13. Do you open your bowels regularly?
14. Do you leak urine when coughing or sneezing?
15. Do you experience any burning or pain when passing urine?
16. What medications are you taking?
17. Do you leak when you cough, sneeze or laugh?

As well as taking a nursing history from the patient, other tests may prove useful.

Mid-stream specimen of urine (MSU)

A clean sample of urine should be obtained and tested with a dip-stick; if the urine is cloudy, offensive smelling or the dip-stick shows positive for blood and/or protein then the urine sample should be sent for microscopy, culture and sensitivity (MC&S). This will demonstrate whether the individual has a urine infection and what types of antibiotics are best to treat it.

The microscopy part of this standard request to the microbiologist involves them examining the urine through a microscope for any debris, casts or blood cells. Any red and/or white blood cells present are counted and a record of the number per mm cubed is made. Urine should not normally contain any cells and a high number of white cells are indicative of an infection. A sample of the urine is then cultured on an agar plate and any bacteria present will grow and can subsequently be identified and reported by the microbiologist. Sometimes a report of mixed flora is received and this implies that the sample was not cleanly taken and there was some contamination – usually from skin. The microbiologist will indicate the significance of any equivocal results.

To obtain a sensitivity profile, the isolated bacteria is grown on another agar plate with small samples of different antibiotics. The micro-biologist is then able to determine which antibiotic will be most effective at clearing the infection and the doctor can make an informed decision regarding a prescription.

Once an individual has finished a course of antibiotics for a urine infection it is always worth sending a further MSU to be tested to ensure that the infection is completely cleared.

Fluid balance charts

These can be useful in giving an indication of input, output, frequency, nocturia and any episodes of incontinence. They can be used with patients at home or in hospital and should be used over a period of at least 48 hours to give an accurate picture of the individual's problems.

In order to gain an exact picture it is also important that charts are filled in accurately and patients should be encouraged to maintain their own charts. The nurse should ensure that the patient understands what is required of them in filling in the charts and what information the team is hoping to gain by so doing. Patients should measure their outputs when possible and if incontinent should indicate this on the chart with an estimate of the volume (e.g. +, ++ or +++).

Residual urine

If it is suspected that an individual is not emptying their bladder fully when voiding, the suspicion must be confirmed and the amount of urine left in the bladder post voiding (i.e. the residual volume) should be ascertained. Ideally this should be done using a bladder scanner, which is a non-invasive technique. The patient is advised to pass urine normally and then asked to lie down and using a bladder scanner, the probe is placed on the skin over the area of the bladder. The bladder scanner works by ultrasound and enables the user to determine the volume of urine present in the bladder.

If a bladder scanner is not available, it may be necessary to pass a temporary catheter after voiding, so measuring the amount of residual urine. This procedure, by its very nature, carries risk of infection and should only be performed if absolutely necessary.

Treatments

Having completed a full assessment of the individual's problems related to elimination, the interdisciplinary team, in consultation with the patient, can plan a management strategy. It is essential that factors which can aggravate bladder problems (see Table 6.1) are treated appropriately, as well as just treating the bladder symptoms. For example, if someone is struggling to get around, an assessment by the physiotherapist may resolve some of the mobility problems allowing the patient to access the toilet more easily and quickly which in turn may result in far fewer episodes of incontinence.

Role of the doctor

Treatment of bladder dysfunction in MS is usually by medication or intermittent self-catheterisation, depending on the outcome of the assessment. The doctor and/or continence nurse can decide on the best way forward.

If a urinary tract infection (UTI) is present it is essential that this is treated and the problems reassessed once the infection is cleared. Urinary tract infections exacerbate symptoms of frequency, urgency and incontinence etc. It is also thought that urinary tract infections can trigger relapses in people with MS and certainly, on an anecdotal level, many people with MS experience a worsening of their disease when a urinary tract infection is present (Metz *et al.*, 1998). Assuming that the MSU was within normal limits and no urinary tract infection is present, the doctor will base treatment on the history given and any residual urine measured. A flow chart detailing the treatment options can be seen in Figure 6.1; this is used in many different centres and can be a useful tool in determining the best course of action for a particular individual.

Medications

Anticholinergic medications are routinely used to treat urgency, frequency and incontinence. Many people with mild to moderate symp-

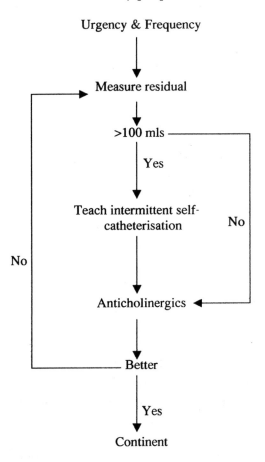

Figure 6.1 Flow chart illustrating recommended treatment of bladder dysfunction. Source: Fowler (1996).

toms will manage well with these alone. They work by blocking contractions of the detrusor muscle and include oxybutynin, detrusitol and propantheline bromide. Tricyclic anti-depressants such as amitriptyline or imipramine may also be helpful. The main side effects of these medications are a dry mouth and throat. The patient can be encouraged to combat this by drinking, sucking mints or boiled sweets. Another option is to freeze tinned pineapple cubes and suck these, which can also provide some relief. Some people are unable to tolerate these side effects and then alternatives should be discussed, such as referral to a continence advisor, urologist or intermittent self-catheterisation.

For people experiencing nocturia, medication such as desmopressin may be used (Eckford *et al.*, 1994). This is available either as a nasal spray or as tablets and is usually taken at night. The effect of desmopressin is to reduce the amount of urine produced and thus it can provide patients with significant relief from nocturia. This in turn can lead to a better night's sleep for both the patient and their partner, and therefore a lessening in fatigue. Patients using desmopressin may also take the medication during the day at times (Hoverd and Fowler, 1998); however, patients should be advised only to take the medication once in every 24 hours.

A very occasional complication of taking desmopressin can be hyponatraemia. The symptoms of hyponatraemia include nausea, headache and feeling generally unwell. If these symptoms occur while taking desmopressin, patients should be advised to contact their GP or MS specialist nurse. A simple blood test to measure serum levels of sodium can be taken and if sodium levels are falling, the patient should be advised against using it in the future.

Contraindications include patients in whom there is doubt as to their compliance (i.e. who may take it more than once in 24 hours – perhaps due to cognitive impairment). It is also best avoided in patients with severe mobility problems and patients with dependent oedema (Hoverd and Fowler, 1998).

The nurse's role

The nurse has a central role to play in assessing the individual's problems and the wider impact of these difficulties as well as in helping the individual to manage the problem. The nurse's skills of tact, empathy, discretion, teaching and support will all be required when working with people with elimination dysfunction.

If the patient is prescribed medication in an attempt to relieve their elimination problems, be it antibiotics, anticholinergics or desmopressin, the nurse must ensure that the patient understands what the medications are hoping to achieve, how to take the medication, potential side effects, and how these can be managed. There is also much the patient can do to help themselves reduce their symptoms and the nurse should take time to explain these to the patient. Some self-help strategies are listed in Table 6.3 and should be self-explanatory.

The nurse should also liaise with other members of the team as necessary.

Some patients may need to use a catheter either via intermittent self-catheterisation or as a long-term solution. The nurse and/or continence advisor and/or MS specialist nurse are vital in teaching and supporting patients and partners in the use and care of catheters and these will be discussed below.

Table 6.3 Self-help strategies for minimising bladder symptoms

- Reduce intake of caffeine, fizzy drinks and alcohol to a minimum (caffeine, carbonated drinks and alcohol all irritate the bladder as well as acting as a mild diuretic)
- Cut down on smoking as this can also irritate the bladder
- Drink at least 2 litres daily. People often find they can drink more water and urinate less frequently as it causes less irritation of the bladder
- Drink 300mls of cranberry juice daily as this can reduce the incidence of infection (Avorn *et al.*, 1994)
- Increase fibre intake to reduce the symptoms of constipation, which can in turn reduce bladder capacity
- Women should be encouraged to do pelvic floor exercises to minimise the risk of stress incontinence (which is unrelated to MS)
- If incomplete emptying and/or frequency is experienced the following technique may be helpful. Once patients feel that they have finished urinating, they should stand up, turn around then sit down and try again. Alternatively applying pressure in the region of the bladder either manually or with a bladder stimulator will often result in the individual passing more urine
- If experiencing recurring urinary tract infection patients should ensure that they are aware of the symptoms (i.e. cloudy urine, offensive odour, burning pain or presence of blood in the urine) and, if any occur, they should take a sample to their GP for testing
- Gentle daily exercise helps to maintain bladder and bowel function
- Ask for help if needed - the contact number for the continence advisors or MS specialist nurse should be supplied
- Patients are often tempted to reduce the amount of fluid drunk each day. Try and avoid this wherever possible and replace cups of tea etc. with water or cordial, which is usually better tolerated

Role of the physiotherapist

The physiotherapists are involved in reducing elimination problems in two ways. Some physiotherapists work specifically with continence issues and can advise patients in much the same way as continence advisors do. The physiotherapists are also vital in addressing any problems with mobility that may be preventing the patients with MS from reaching the toilet in time.

Role of the occupational therapist

The occupational therapist can look at various issues in the home to enable easier access to the toilet. They may recommend that a downstairs toilet is fitted or provide aids to allow the individual to get upstairs more easily. They may provide a urinal for use overnight and can assess the need for grab rails, raised toilet seats etc. to improve access and increase independence for people with MS. Occupational therapists may also be able to advise people on suitable clothing etc., making the process of actually going to the toilet easier.

Role of the dietician

The dietician can advise the patient on an appropriate diet to minimise problems of constipation. This can aggravate urinary dysfunction by reducing bladder capacity as the bowel stretches due to the storage of constipated stool.

Role of the continence advisor

The continence advisor is a specialist nurse dealing specifically with bladder and bowel dysfunction. They are often community based although some hospitals may have access to a continence advisor for inpatients.

Their role is in assessing the nature of the problem and advising the GP/doctor on appropriate medication. They also teach the patients how to manage the problem themselves and will teach intermittent self-catheterisation, catheter care etc. as required. The continence advisors are an excellent resource for patients and their families as well as the health care team involved in the patient's care.

Intermittent self-catheterisation

Intermittent self-catheterisation (ISC) is the technique of passing a catheter into the bladder, drawing off the urine, and then removing the catheter again. Ideally patients are taught to do this themselves, occasionally it may be necessary for their partner or carer to perform intermittent catheterisation for them.

ISC is indicated when someone is suffering from incomplete emptying which results in frequency, urgency and often incontinence, the benefits can be many (see Table 6.4).

Many patients are initially guarded in their response to the suggestion of using ISC. However most people find it relatively easy and it can have a hugely positive impact on their quality of life (Webb *et al.*, 1990).

> I can go out now without having to carry a spare pair of knickers or worrying about where the nearest toilet is. Using the catheters is quite easy once you get used to it and has made a huge difference to both our lives.
>
> (BD – part-time florist and wife to GD talking about using ISC)

The nature of the technique is intimate. Teaching someone how to self-catheterise must be approached with sensitivity and should not be rushed.

The reason for using ISC, and the hoped for benefits of using the technique, should be explored fully with the patient before starting. The basics of the technique should also be explained to ensure the patient understands that the technique is neither painful nor too difficult. Prior to showing the patient how to self-catheterise, it is important that they are familiar with their own anatomy. Clear diagrams and a mirror are essential and the time needed to be spent on this aspect of training should be assessed on an individual basis. Some people will already be familiar with their anatomy and comfortable with themselves, while others may find even using the mirror to identify parts of their anatomy very uncomfort-

Table 6.4 The benefits of using intermittent self-catheterisation

---

- Reduces incidence of urinary tract infection
- Improves continence
- Puts patient in control, enhancing independence, self-esteem and quality of life (Hunt *et al.*, 1996)
- Reduces symptoms of frequency and urgency
- Allows people to leave their house unconcerned about the site of the nearest toilet
- Improves confidence
- May result in reduced levels of fatigue

---

able. In order to use ISC successfully people must have a certain degree of ease with their own bodies and this may take some time to acquire.

Teaching female self-catheterisation

1. Assemble the equipment needed: mirror, catheter, wipes or soap and water, dry towel and a bowl to collect the urine if not catheterising over the toilet.
2. Wash hands with soap and water.
3. Position self comfortably, thighs need to be spaced apart. Once familiar with the technique it is often easiest to sit on the toilet, or on a chair next to the toilet.
4. Lubricate catheter; some catheters come ready lubricated, and patients should be advised appropriately depending on the type of catheter used.
5. The catheter should be inserted into the urethra until the urine begins to flow. The catheter can then be inserted further in until the bladder is fully drained.
6. Once the urine has stopped flowing the catheter should be withdrawn slowly, if more urine begins to flow then the withdrawal should be stopped, until urine flow stops once more. This should be repeated until the catheter is withdrawn.
7. Reusing the catheter depends on the type of catheter and individual circumstances and should be discussed when the catheters are supplied.

Male catheterisation

1. Assemble the equipment needed: catheter, wipes or soap and water, dry towel and a bowl to collect the urine if not catheterising over a toilet.
2. Wash hands with soap and water.
3. Position self comfortably.
4. Lubricate catheter as instructed. Larger catheters are needed for male catheterisation and a longer length of catheter should be lubricated.
5. Hold penis straight up from body and insert catheter into the urethra until the urine begins to flow.
6. Once the urine has stopped flowing the catheter should be withdrawn slowly, if more urine begins to flow then the withdrawal should be stopped, until urine flow stops once more. This should be repeated until the catheter is withdrawn.

7. Reusing the catheter depends on the type of catheter and individual circumstances and should be discussed when the catheters are supplied.

Frequency of ISC

Essentially this is determined on an individual basis. However, most people catheterise themselves between two-four times daily. Once adept at self-catheterisation, patients can use the technique while out and about. This can free people from the need to remain near a toilet or return home frequently and can lead to an improved quality of life for the whole family.

Most people manage well with ISC but some people do find it more difficult than others do, for example, if they have dexterity problems in their hands or suffer from frequent spasms. The nature of MS also means that people's needs can change over time. Due to these potential problems it is essential that patients be given ongoing support and a telephone number to use if problems occur (e.g. the district nurse or continence advisor).

Long-term catheters

Urethral catheterisation may be short-term or long-term but should only be used in intractable incontinence when all other measures have been tried and found to be ineffective (Doherty and Winder, 2000).

Indwelling catheters can be left connected to a drainage bag to allow free drainage or they can be fitted with a valve to allow intermittent drainage, which ensures some retention of bladder tone.

Prior to fitting an indwelling catheter, the pros and cons of having a catheter for the individual should be discussed fully with them, their family and members of the interdisciplinary team who are involved in their case.

Long-term use of an indwelling catheter can lead to complications. These include urinary tract infection, blockage, bypassing, irritation and trauma.

Urine infections

Organisms can be introduced into the bladder via the catheter during insertion. Organisms may also migrate through the interior of the catheter tube from the drainage system.

Patients and carers should be taught how to care for their catheter. Nurses emptying patients' bags and (dis)connecting drainage bags should ensure they always use aseptic technique. The outlet tap has been shown to be at significant risk of infection from peoples' hands (Wilson and Coates, 1996). Alcohol wipes are known to be ineffective for cleaning the taps and single use disposable gloves are recommended instead which should be changed between patients. The risk of infection increases in proportion to the length of time the catheter is in situ.

Trauma

Trauma can be caused by the catheter being insufficiently supported resulting in the catheter balloon straining the bladder neck and/or the urethra. In extreme cases the urethral meatus may become eroded leading to a split in the penile head or the labia.

When a leg bag is being worn this should be supported by the Velcro straps provided or often more effectively, by a piece of stockinet fitted around both the leg and the catheter bag. This not only ensures that it is kept secure but also keeps the bag as discreet as possible.

Overnight the night drainage bag can be attached to the leg bag. This gives sufficient slack in the system to allow the patient to move in bed. The potential for trauma can be further reduced by securing the catheter tube to the top of the thigh with some tape. The advisability of this depends largely on skin integrity and should be decided on an individual basis.

Catheter blockage

This can be caused by several different factors which include:

- kinking of the drainage tube;
- excess mucous accumulating around the drainage hole;
- the bladder wall being sucked into the drainage holes;
- displacement of the catheter into the urethra;
- constipation resulting in pressure on the urethra and catheter hole and crystal formation (if pH value is greater than 7.2) (after Doherty and Winder, 2000).

If a catheter continues to block, bladder washouts can be useful. The catheter must be changed as often as is necessary. The desired frequency of catheter change is every three months; however, some individuals are unable to tolerate a catheter for this length of time. This should be accepted and the catheter changed as often as necessary for each individual. The emergency situation of a catheter blocking in the community should be avoided as far as possible by pre-empting potential problems.

Bypassing

This is said to occur when urine leaks around the catheter tube rather than draining through the tube itself. It can occur secondary to a blocked catheter tube or alternatively it may occur as a result of bladder spasms. It is not recommended that the size of catheter is changed in response to bypassing but rather that anticholinergic medication is used to prevent further spasms (Namey, 1997).

Supra pubic catheters

These are inserted into the bladder via the abdominal wall. The initial insertion is a surgical procedure. Supra pubic catheters are indicated if a long-term catheter is required. They are generally preferable to a urethral catheter as patients often consider them to be less intrusive, (particularly if they are sexually active) and more easily managed. They are not without their complications, however, and full discussion with a consultant urologist prior to the insertion is required. It is also essential that patients be supported following the procedure for as long as is necessary. Potential complications include delayed healing and over granulation at the insertion site as well as those listed for urethral catheters.

It is important to note that most patients with bladder dysfunction are able to manage their symptoms with self-help techniques and possibly medication. The need for ISC is less common and the use of an indwelling catheter tends to be a last resort but may provide relief from uncomfortable and embarrassing symptoms for the individual when indicated.

Bowel symptoms in MS

Normal bowel function

The bowel receives the food and liquid eaten and drunk by the individual. Nutrients are absorbed and waste products are retained within the bowel. The waste products are later eliminated in the form of faeces. As the large bowel fills with faeces, the stretch receptors stimulate the cerebral cortex (via S2–S4) and the urge to defecate is felt. If the individual does not wish to defecate at that time voluntary control is exerted on the external sphincter to keep it closed until such time as defecation is appropriate. Once the individual wishes to defecate the external sphincter is relaxed and the individual 'bears down'. This is known as the Valsalva manoeuvre and occurs as the individual takes a deep breath and tries to breathe out while maintaining a closed glottis. This causes an increase in abdominal pressure assisting defecation. The area of the spinal chord T6 –T12 must be intact to enable someone to bear down in this way.

Approximately 60% of people with MS will experience bowel dysfunction at some stage of their disease (Namey, 1997). By far the most common problem is constipation; however, occasionally people also suffer from faecal incontinence. Understandably faecal incontinence is by far the most distressing complaint and has a huge impact if it occurs. Unfortunately faecal incontinence is also much harder to treat than constipation.

Constipation

This is said to occur when someone does not open their bowels as often as they are used to, and/or if the stools produced are hard and lumpy, and the individual has difficulty evacuating the stool. Everybody has a different frequency of defecation that is normal for them. This can vary from two-three times a day to once weekly and this should be borne in mind when assessing an individual.

The causes of constipation can be many:

- reduced fluid intake (often in response to elimination dysfunction);
- low fibre intake;
- reduced activity (may be unavoidable in MS);
- medication (e.g. codeine, anticholinergics);
- demyelination of the sacral area leading to a sluggish bowel;
- weakened abdominal muscles causing difficulty in bearing down;
- reduced sensation so that the urge to defecate is not felt.

The nurse must assess the patients' normal bowel habit, diet, fluid intake, appearance of stool, accessibility of toilet and privacy (or otherwise) of toilet.

The individual themselves can often make simple changes to their lifestyle which can improve their bowel movement. The nurse is responsible for assessing their relevance and for explaining the importance of these simple interventions to the patient, i.e.

- Patients should aim to drink at least two litres of fluid daily (preferably not caffeine or carbonated).
- Patients should increase the amount of fibre in their diet. Fresh fruit and vegetables can be enjoyed as can eating ready-to-eat dried fruits. Using a high-fibre breakfast cereal and adding fibre to foods such as yoghurts, custard etc. can also help.
- Patients should increase activity levels if possible.
- Patients should try and establish a routine to their bowel movements. Most people find it easiest to open their bowels about half an hour after a meal when the gastrocolic reflex is strongest, particularly in a morning.

If these measures are insufficient then laxatives may be used. Laxatives work in different ways and should be chosen to meet the needs of the individual:

- bulk formers e.g. bran, methylcellulose;
- stool softeners, e.g. Docusate;
- stimulants to promote bowel activity, e.g. senna and bisacodyl;
- osmotic agents (draw water into the stool to act as a softener), e.g. Lactulose.

There are many laxatives on the market and the choice should be made according to local policy, individual need and ease of use.

Occasionally constipation may not be relieved by laxatives in which case suppositories may be required. These stimulate the bowel as well as providing lubrication of the stool. They may be used in conjunction with other laxatives. Suppositories can be used either routinely (though preferably not daily) or more usually, once or twice weekly.

Enemas may be used if all else fails but routine use should be avoided if at all possible as the bowel may become dependent on them, and not work without them.

It is important to establish a routine. This may take some time and is often a matter of trial and error initially. The support and advice of a nurse (e.g. district nurse, practice nurse, continence advisor or MS specialist nurse) is essential to the development of an effective bowel programme.

Faecal incontinence

This is perhaps one of the most distressing and socially inhibiting symptoms that can occur in MS. Fortunately it is quite rare although this is cold comfort to those people experiencing it. There can be a number of causes:

- overflow due to impaction;
- diarrhoea due to too much fibre or overuse of laxatives;
- diarrhoea due to a gastrointestinal virus unrelated to MS;
- poor sphincter control;
- hyper-reflexic bowel.

A full assessment should be made including a review of recent history of bowel movements (i.e. has there been any change?), diet, fluid intake, medications, frequency of the problem, any associated pain or discomfort and any alteration in anal sensation.

Due to the upsetting nature of this symptom it is essential that the nurse proceed with as much tact and empathy as possible. It is also important that the nurse reassures the patient and their partner (if appropriate) that these symptoms are likely to be due to the MS and that they are not the only ones to have experienced these symptoms.

Once the assessment is complete, interventions to alleviate the problem may become obvious e.g. reducing excessive laxative use or relieving impaction. However, if the problem is caused by demyelination of the spinal cord resulting in loss of sphincter control or hyper-reflexia, other interventions may be required.

As with any bowel problem it is important to try and establish a routine. If the individual can ensure their bowels are emptied each morning (using the gastrocolic reflex to maximise success) this may minimise the chance of involuntary evacuation during the day. It may also be useful to use a suppository initially to assist in establishing a routine and ensuring the bowels are emptied. If the bowel is hyper-reflexive, i.e. going into spasms in the same way the bladder can, then anticholinergic medication can help (Namey, 1997).

It may be necessary to prescribe a bowel inhibitor such as immodium or loperamide for use when the patient wishes to go out. Their continued or regular use, however, is not recommended as this can lead to impaction/constipation that can exacerbate the problem.

When someone suffers from faecal incontinence it is essential that attention is paid to skin integrity and great care is taken to ensure the skin remains clean and dry. People should not be left sitting in soiled pads etc. and carers must be made aware of this. It is vital that appropriate help and advice is sought immediately a problem is noted. Establishing an effective regime to combat faecal incontinence often takes time and can prove very disheartening to the patient and their family. The ongoing support of a nurse is essential. If different regimes are tried without success, referral to a gastroenterologist should be considered.

The ultimate goal is for the individual to move their bowels regularly, without discomfort and in a setting that is appropriate, comfortable and private so maintaining their independence and dignity.

CHAPTER 7

Sexuality and pregnancy

Introduction

The concept of sexuality and of sex itself is far more complex than just being able to have intercourse. Sexuality is an integral aspect of every individual and may be defined as an awareness of one's body as a source of pleasure, a sense of self as a sexual being and a vision of self as a male or female (Few, 1993). It is everyone's right that they should be able to enjoy a state of sexual health, regardless of age, illness and disability (Weston, 1993).

People with MS report a high incidence of sexual dysfunction; figures vary from about 50% to as high as 91% (see Table 7.1). These reports tend to focus largely on physical problems such as erectile dysfunction, loss of libido and reduced sensation; the wider impact of MS on an individual's sexuality is often overlooked.

Table 7.1 Reported incidence of sexual dysfunction

Male erectile dysfunction	70-80%	Eardley and Sethia,
Male loss of libido	>50%	1998b
Change in sexual function in		
Men with advanced disease	91%	Benson, 1997
Females with sexual difficulties	56-72%	Lilius et al., 1976

Sexual dysfunction can have a number of causes. Primary sexual dysfunction is caused directly by demyelination within the central nervous system (e.g. numbness in the peri-anal area). Secondary sexual dysfunction occurs as a direct result of symptoms of MS, e.g. spasticity or incontinence. Tertiary sexual dysfunction occurs as a result of the psychosocial impact of MS, e.g. depression, changing roles between partners etc. (Foley and

Sanders, 1997). It is often a combination of different factors that ultimately cause problems (see Table 7.2 for further examples).

Table 7.2 Factors that may impact on sexual dysfunction in people with MS

Primary sexual dysfunction:	Reduced peri-anal sensation
	Other medical conditions (e.g. diabetes)
	Inability to maintain erection
	Inability to achieve orgasm
Secondary sexual dysfunction:	Fatigue
	Continence problems
	Spasticity
	Pain
	Sensory problems
Tertiary sexual dysfunction:	Low self-esteem
	Poor body image
	Role changes within the relationship
	Depression
	Stress
	Unrealistic expectations
Iatrogenic:	Medications (e.g. amitriptylline, carbamazepine)
	Smoking
	Excessive alcohol intake
	Age
	Use of cannabis or other recreational drugs

Everyone's sexuality is influenced by many factors such as culture, personality, upbringing, religion etc. and evolves throughout our lifespan in response to these factors. The impact of an illness such as MS on definition, expression and experience of sexuality can be significant. Dividing the causes of sexual dysfunction into primary, secondary and tertiary can be a useful technique to employ when assessing someone who is complaining of sexual difficulties; not least because it provides a useful model to ensure a holistic approach to care is used.

This chapter will review the potential problems faced by people with MS and the treatment options available. The impact of other symptoms on an individual's sexuality will be explored and the role of the nurse in this context examined at length. The chapter will conclude with a review of pregnancy and MS.

Assessment

As with any symptom in MS a thorough assessment of the problem(s) must be made. The aim of the assessment is initially to determine the cause of any difficulties experienced.

A full medical and neurological evaluation and sexual history should be taken, preferably with the patient's partner present if both wish it. The assessment needs to be made in a sensitive manner and requires a health care professional with a thorough knowledge of sexual dysfunction in MS and who feels comfortable discussing such intimate issues. While the nurse is not always the best person to undertake this detailed assessment (see below); they may often be the health care professional who realises that the person with MS is having sexual problems. The nurse can then ensure that the patient is managed appropriately by the relevant member of the interdisciplinary team.

Primary sexual dysfunction in men

In men, primary sexual dysfunction is most typically manifested as erectile dysfunction. Nervous impulses travel between the central nervous system and the penis which are responsible for initiating and maintaining an erection. When the appropriate nervous impulse is received in response to sexual stimulus, the arterial blood flow to the penis increases. This increase in blood flow combined with the expansion of the penile tissues compresses venous outflow resulting in an erection.

The spinal cord contains the nerve pathways to and from the genitals; in particular these areas are S2–S4 and T10–L2 (Benson, 1997). It should be noted that these areas of the spinal cord are also closely involved in the control of elimination. If someone is complaining of elimination problems, the chances are high that they are also experiencing some degree of sexual dysfunction.

There are many different options available to treat erectile dysfunction. These range from oral medication to surgical implantation of a prosthesis.

Oral medication

There are a number of medications that can be given orally that may have some sort of positive influence on erectile dysfunction. The most recent and possibly most well known is sildenafil (Viagra). Taking sildenafil does not automatically result in an erection; however, if erotic or sexual stimulation is experienced, erectile function is enabled. Sildenafil is not an aphrodisiac and has no effect on sexual drive or libido, rather it enables normal erectile physiology (Eardley and Sethia, 1998c). A trial studying 178 males with spinal cord injury demonstrated a significant improvement in both erection and sexual intercourse when using sildenafil (Holmgren *et al.*, 1998).

The response to sildenafil is dose related. Most men will find a dose of 50mg or 100mg effective. If higher doses are used then side effects become more problematical. In the UK sildenafil is licensed to treat sexual dysfunction in men only. It is not as yet widely available on prescription; however, men with MS are one of the categories of patient allowed to obtain sildenafil via a GP prescription.

If someone is prescribed sildenafil they should be advised to take 50mg initially about one hour prior to intercourse. The dose can be titrated up or down (25–100mg) depending on the individual's response. Potential side effects include headache, flushing and dizziness, a few patients also complain of dyspepsia. It is important that patients taking medication containing nitrates of any kind (e.g. glycerol trinitrate prescribed for angina) must *not* take sildenafil as it can negate the effect of the nitrate containing medication.

While sildenafil is now the treatment of choice, there are still other options available for men who either do not respond or are unable to tolerate it.

Intraurethral medication

It is easier for medications to be absorbed via the urethral mucosa rather than the penile skin. Medication entering the body via this route will easily be able to access the smooth muscle of the corpus cavernosa via the extensive venous network.

This mode of entry is used by the MUSE(tm) system. MUSE(tm) stands for 'medicated urethral system for erection' and delivers prostaglandins in pellet form via the urethra.

The patient is asked to void a small amount of urine initially, as a few drops of urine help the pellet to dissolve. The medication is supplied with a specially designed administration device and this is inserted fully into the urethra (about 3cm). There is a button at the end of the device, which is then depressed, so delivering the pellet into the urethra. Once the pellet is administered and the delivery device removed, the patient (or their partner) is advised to massage the penis for several minutes. The patient should also be advised to avoid lying down for 10–15 minutes to gain the most from the medication.

The dose is variable (from 125 to 1000 micrograms) and should be titrated to suit the individual. The patient can expect an erection to develop within about 15 minutes and last for between 30 and 60 minutes. Some people find that using a constriction ring placed around the base of the penis prior to using the MUSE™ system can improve the strength and duration of their erection. Studies have not shown spectacular results but have shown a significant improvement when compared with placebo (Padma-Nathan *et al.*, 1997). However, this remains a very useful second line treatment.

Side effects tend to occur in about one-third of people using it (according to the above study) but are mild. The most common effect tends to be penile pain with occasional mild urethral trauma. Partners may occasionally experience vaginal discomfort and itching. Despite these problems, the treatment is usually well tolerated. The effect of prostaglandin in the ejaculate on pregnant women has not been studied in any depth, however as prostaglandins are used in pessary form to induce labour, it is recommended that MUSE™ is not used by men whose partners are pregnant.

Intracorporeal injections

Injecting a medication to induce an erection into the corpus cavernosum has been used since the 1980s. There are different types of medication available for injection. Prostaglandin is widely used in the UK and Europe with a mixture of prostaglandin, papaverine and phentolamine (known as trimix) used largely in America.

As with transurethral administration, the prostaglandin produces an erection by acting on the smooth muscle within the penis. To date prostaglandin is the safest and most effective of the agents available (Eardley and Sethia, 1998a).

Prostaglandin is unstable in liquid form and must be mixed prior to use and stored at cool temperatures. Once mixed and drawn into the syringe, the solution is injected into the penile shaft. The patient (or the patient's partner) should then massage the penis for about 30 seconds. In a suitable individual an erection will develop within 5–10 minutes.

It is beyond the scope of this book to explain the technique of penile self-injection in any length. However, needless to say, the patient and their partner will often need a great deal of support and education to use this technique successfully and a nurse with specialist knowledge of the procedure is often central in providing this support.

Patients with neurogenic erectile dysfunction are particularly sensitive to injection therapy; however, the dose can be titrated to suit the individual. Patients should be advised that the erection does not disappear on ejaculation but often persists for 1–2 hours. If the erection persists for more than 4 hours, they should be advised to attend the clinic or accident and emergency department as priapism may develop. Priapism is an erection that persists for more than 4 hours and has the potential to cause ischaemic damage. Priapism in this context can be easily resolved by giving the patient oral terbutaline (5–10mg); this can be prescribed in clinic and taken home by the patient with full instructions as to when and how to take it if required.

The success rate for prostaglandin injection has been shown to be approximately 70% (Junemann *et al.*, 1996). Potential side effects include penile pain and bruising, less commonly hypotension or urethral bleeding may occur. Fibrosis of the corpus cavernosum may develop with long-term use although the risk of this with prostaglandin is low.

Vacuum devices

There are still some patients for whom oral, transurethral or intracorporeal medications are unsuitable and/or ineffective. In this instance they may well benefit from using a vacuum device.

For men who can achieve an erection but have difficulty maintaining it, a constriction ring placed around the base of the penis once erection has occurred may be sufficient. This works by preventing venous drainage from the penis, so maintaining the erection until the ring is removed.

Most men, however, will need to use a constriction ring in conjunction with a vacuum device. There are many different types of vacuum devices available. Each consists of three main sections: a clear cylinder which is placed over the penis and which forms an airtight seal against the pubis; a pump mechanism used to create the vacuum and a constriction ring. This is fitted to the base of the penis once erection is achieved so maintaining erection and allowing easy removal of the vacuum device.

The majority of men can use a vacuum device with figures as high as 92% of people achieving an erection reported (Witherington, 1989). However, the vacuum device does require good manual dexterity which can be a problem for people with MS. If this is the case their partner may be able to apply the device for them. Other potential problems include loss of angle of erection, bruising, discoloration, difficulty ejaculating and a drop in penile temperature, which may be uncomfortable for the partner.

In summary there are many different treatments available for men with primary sexual dysfunction as a result of MS. The first line treatment must be oral medication, if the patient cannot tolerate this or does not respond, the alternatives should be discussed with the patient and their partner at some length and the most appropriate second line treatment for that individual decided.

Primary sexual dysfunction in women

Studies looking at the sexual difficulties of women with MS are few and far between and most have problematical methodology. Sample sizes are too small, control groups are omitted and sample populations are not representative of the MS community (Foley and Sanders, 1997a).

A methodologically sound survey (McCabe *et al.*, 1996) showed that a total of 79.6% of women reported at least one problem (see Table 7.3). Despite this over half of the sample reported no undue concerns about their sexual difficulties.

Assessment of women with sexual problems should be made in the same way as for men. Women too will have complex and multi-layered problems with primary, secondary and tertiary symptoms impacting on sexual function. Primary sexual dysfunction in women can take many different forms, e.g. reduced libido, reduced genital sensation, reduced frequency and/or intensity of orgasm.

Unfortunately treatments for women with sexual dysfunction are less well developed than those for men. This said, problems such as poor vaginal lubrication can be easily solved by using a water-based lubricant (e.g. K-Y jelly).

Altered sensation in the genital area may respond to medications such as tegretol or amitriptyline the same way as altered sensation elsewhere in the body. Reduced genital sensation is more difficult to remedy. Some women find that using vibrators or other sexual aids can be helpful, stimulation by their partner may also increase the intensity of the sensation. Mail order companies can be a useful resource when selecting sexual aids.

Table 7.3 Problems with sexual function reported by women with MS

Lack of sexual interest	29%
Failure to achieve orgasm	23.7%
Poor lubrication	19.4%
Reduced satisfaction with masturbation	9.7%
Painful intercourse	6.5%
Vaginismus	1.1%

Loss of desire is possibly the most difficult problem to counter. Reduced libido is often a result of secondary (e.g. fatigue) or tertiary (e.g. low self-esteem) symptoms and as such may improve once the root cause is successfully tackled.

Some women still experience sexual pleasure although their desire to participate in intercourse is lost. With open communication between themselves and their partner, this problem can be compensated for (Foley and Sanders, 1997a).

There are no large-scale trials of medications to improve desire etc. among women with MS. Sometimes medications such as testosterone, yohimbine or even sildenafil (NB this is not licensed for use in women at present) may be helpful. However from anecdotal reports, the effectiveness of these medications tends to be moderate at best. Any medications such as those mentioned are best prescribed under the auspices of a specialist sexual health clinic.

Secondary sexual dysfunction in men and women

This occurs as a result of other MS symptoms impacting on sexual function. Treatment of the symptom in question will often resolve the resulting sexual problems. For example one of the most commonly occurring MS symptoms that has a direct effect on sexuality is fatigue (Valleroy and Kraft, 1984). If the fatigue can be managed successfully then sexual function should improve. Other strategies that can be employed by the couple include resting prior to sexual activity; changing the timing of sexual activity to coincide with the MS partner's 'best time' and adopting less tiring positions. Again open communication about the nature of the problem between partners is essential to avoid misunderstandings and the potential for building resentment.

Bladder and bowel dysfunctions are another common factor that can cause secondary sexual dysfunction. If a woman with MS is taking anticholinergic medication (e.g. oxybutynin or detrusitol), they may find that the vagina becomes very dry. This can be overcome by using a water based lubricating gel. In men these same medications can sometimes interfere with erectile function (Crenshaw and Goldberg, 1996). In these circumstances it may be appropriate for the patient to modify their medication schedules, in consultation with their doctor or MS specialist nurse, to minimise any potential problems.

Both men and women may fear leakage of urine during sexual activity. Cutting down on fluids prior to having intercourse may help, as may emptying the bladder just prior to any sexual activity.

Sometimes bladder problems may mean that the individual needs to use a urethral catheter; however, this need not be a bar to sexual activity. A man can disconnect the catheter from the drainage bag and spigot the end. By folding the catheter tube back along the penile shaft and using a condom over the whole, the physical barrier of the catheter can be overcome. Women can also disconnect the catheter and place a spigot in the end of the tube. The catheter tube can then be moved to one side and taped out of the way. Various positions for the tube can be tried to find one that both partners find comfortable.

It cannot be stressed how important it is for partners to communicate with each other about fears, anxieties and the problems each may encounter.

Sometimes people with MS experience areas of altered sensation. These can be anywhere in the body and may be experienced as painful, hypersensitive to touch or numbness. It can be useful in these circumstances for the partner to explore the person's body gently in order to determine which areas respond pleasurably to touch and which areas are best avoided (a technique sometimes called body mapping).

MS can cause changes in attention span and the ability to concentrate. This may result in the person with MS appearing to lose interest during sexual activity. Understandably this is often particularly off-putting for their partner who may interpret the apparent lack of interest as feeling unloved and undesirable. Again, understanding of the problem by both partners is vital. Creating an atmosphere that is conducive to sexual activity and developing strategies that allow the partner with MS to focus once more on the intimacy they are sharing with their partner, can be helpful. Humour can be used in this context but should only be used sensitively and within the safe confines of a close relationship.

Tertiary sexual dysfunction in men and women

Tertiary sexual dysfunction is that caused by the psychosocial aspect of MS. People with MS often have low self-confidence – 'If I can't even make my body do what I want, how can anyone else expect anything of me.' Body image also tends to be low, people may be unable to wear the clothes or shoes they would like to, they may find it difficult to style their hair or apply make-up in the way they would like etc. In addition, people with MS may also require walking aids and other aids and adaptations around the house, including the bedroom. This can result in people feeling distinctly unsexy.

Another factor that can have an impact at a tertiary level is the role change that can occur within the relationship as a result of MS. The person with MS may no longer be able to contribute to the relationship in the same way e.g. they may no longer be the main wage earner or they may not be able to shop and clean. Some people may find that they may have to rely on their partner to perform intimate cares such as intermittent self-catheterisation or assistance with bathing, which transforms their partner from lover to carer and these two roles can be difficult to switch between for both partners. Having other family members or social service carers take over the intimate personal cares can be one solution. Alternatively separating caring tasks from romantic times both in terms of time of day and environment can be helpful.

The effect on the partner

The effect on the partner of someone with MS who has sexual difficulties is often overlooked but can be profound. It has been shown that change in sexual function is the most significant indicator of relationship dissatisfaction (Chandler and Brown, 1998). People with MS have a higher rate of divorce than people without MS and it is likely that sexual dysfunction is a significant contributor to this. As can be seen from the information above, there is often much that can be done to help relieve or manage sexual dysfunction. The most difficult step for people to take is to ask for help in the first place and it is often the role of the nurse to address these issues in the first instance.

The role of the nurse

The vast majority of health professionals, including nurses, find that broaching the subject of sexual dysfunction can be very difficult; as a result many choose not to do so.

As nurses we can talk at length to people about their bladder and bowel problems without feeling awkward or embarrassed and our approach towards addressing any sexual problems should initially at least, be equally matter of fact. Each nurse will develop his or her own style and own way of introducing the subject, the important point is that the subject is broached. Although the nurse may not have the knowledge base to advise the patient directly, they should always be aware of who to refer the patient to in order that they can access appropriate advice and treatment (e.g. consultant neurologist, consultant urologist, MS specialist nurse, local sexual health clinic). The rest of this chapter examines the problems experienced by nurses and other health professionals in addressing these issues and suggests some strategies that may help.

A model to facilitate discussion of sexual dysfunction

One of the most commonly used models and perhaps one of the most useful is known as P-LI-SS-IT (Anon, 1976). This model operates on a series of different levels and the nurse can choose whichever level is appropriate for them depending on their own experience, knowledge base and comfort in discussing sexuality.

Level 1: Permission (P)

This is the most basic level and one that all nurses should be able to achieve. It requires the nurse to create a comfortable, safe environment to enable the person with MS to discuss any concerns they may have about their sexuality and/or sexual function.

Basic counselling skills such as the use of reflection and open-ended questions can encourage the person with MS to discuss sensitive issues that may be troubling them. It is often necessary for the nurse to use cue questions so that the individual understands it is acceptable for them to discuss any sexual problems if they so wish (i.e. giving permission).

If the patient chooses to discuss any problems they are having with the nurse, the nurse must discuss these in a non-judgemental way and reassure the person with MS wherever necessary, that their problems are relatively common and that any sexual experimentation to over-come these problems is appropriate. The nurse should also ensure that suitable information leaflets are available and should know how to access further help and support for the person with MS if necessary (RCN, 2000).

Level 2: Limited information (LI)

To work at this level the nurse should have sufficient knowledge of the potential problems to provide the person with MS with limited informa-tion relating to sexuality. For example the nurse may discuss the possibil-ity of erectile dysfunction with a man who is complaining of bladder problems, as they know that the two are often associated.

Level 3: Specific suggestions (SS)

To function at this level of the model, nurses need to have a specialist knowledge base with respect to sexual function related to MS. Specific suggestions to help people cope with the problems they are experiencing are made.

Level 4: Intensive therapy (IT)

This level involves the nurse dealing with complex interpersonal and psychological issues with patients who have specific sexual and relationship problems. Any nurse operating at this level will have specialist training in this area of nursing (RCN, 2000).

It goes without saying that any discussion of sexuality should be undertaken in a suitable environment, i.e. in a quiet room where privacy and no interruptions are assured. Before embarking on a discussion of sexual problems in any depth, the nurse should ensure that this is what the person with MS and their partner want. Sometimes a couple may not have had intercourse for a considerable length of time but may be perfectly happy with this, the idea of restoring sexual function to the affected partner may completely alter the balance of the relationship. It is also important that the nurse does not assume all patients are heterosexual or have the same attitudes and values as themselves. Nurses should also always demonstrate respect of different cultures and religious backgrounds.

Discussing sexuality can be a very difficult thing to do and it is vital that the nurse themselves feel comfortable exploring these issues. To this end the nurse should be well supported by their colleagues and appropriate members of the interdisciplinary team.

Pregnancy in MS

Historically women with MS were advised not to get pregnant, as it was believed this would cause a significant increase in the mother's level of disability. As the peak age range for diagnosis of MS is almost the same as for childbirth, this advice caused severe distress to many couples. It is now known that this belief is unfounded and advice to women with MS wishing to get pregnant today is very different.

A multi-centre European study of pregnancy in MS demonstrated that the rate of relapse during pregnancy decreases (Confavreux et al., 1998). They also demonstrated that disease activity as shown by MRI scanning was reduced, particularly during the third trimester of pregnancy. However the study also reported a significant increase in relapses in the first few months post-natally which gradually returns to the individual's normal risk of relapse about 12 months after the birth. Another study examined the long-term effects of pregnancy on prognosis in MS and found that there was a reduced risk of developing a progressive course in women who became pregnant after the onset of their MS (Runmarker and Anderson, 1995). That they concluded there was a better prognosis for pregnant women may be confounded by the methodology used. They compared two groups of women with MS (matched for neurological deficit), one group became pregnant and the others did not. It may be that the choice of whether or not to become pregnant was influenced by the woman's experience to date of her MS. Thus those women experiencing more problems would be less likely to choose to become pregnant. However, whether or not a better prognosis for women with MS who become pregnant can be assured, the study certainly did not demonstrate any long-term worsening of the disease as a result of pregnancy; a conclusion which is confirmed by most authors (Kalb and LaRocca, 1997).

Pre-conception

Contraception

Women with MS have more reason than most to plan their pregnancies carefully and to this end, contraception is important. There is no evidence that contraception has any impact on the disease process in MS (Thorogood and Hannaford, 1998). Therefore advice to people with MS regarding family planning need be no different than for anyone else, although a review of medication is needed as described below.

Effect of pregnancy on MS

Before a couple with MS choose to get pregnant there are often many questions that they wish to discuss with their doctor or nurse. They may have heard that MS is worsened by pregnancy and will need reassurance on this point. It is also important that the expectations of the couple regarding the birth and post-natal period are explored. While statistically pregnancy has no effect on the long-term course of the disease, the majority of women will experience some degree of relapse in the first few months after the birth. The couple should be aware of this and encouraged to explore the implications of having a relapse with a young baby for them as a couple.

While the statistics show no long-term effects on MS due to pregnancy, it must be made clear that these are statistics and as with most things in MS, there can be no certainty as to the outcome for any given individual. There are instances of women who have developed profoundly disabling relapses post-natally and who have made only a partial recovery. These instances are very much the exception and there is no way of knowing whether or not the individual would have experienced an equally disabling relapse if they had not become pregnant. The likelihood of the pregnancy making no long-term difference to the woman's disease course should be emphasised. Occasionally, the prospective father in particular may have concerns about his partner that outweigh his desire for a child. The couple should be encouraged to explore any fears and concerns together.

Risk of passing on MS to the child

Couples also often ask about the risk of passing on MS to their child. While MS is not hereditary, there is a genetic component and the risk for the child of someone with MS developing the disease themselves is higher than that of someone with no MS in the family. The risk for someone with a first-degree relative with MS is approximately 3% rather than the 0.01% risk quoted for people with no relatives with MS (Sadovnick et al., 1988). It should be stressed that this is a small risk and future developments both in terms of treating symptoms and of disease modifying therapies should not be discounted when considering the risks involved.

On the practical side, the couple should be encouraged to plan for the post-natal period which will be very tiring at best. Planning before the birth to enlist help from family and friends afterwards is essential to ensure that the person with MS gets sufficient rest and sleep.

Medication

There are some medications used to treat symptoms of MS which should be stopped prior to conception if possible. Women should be strongly advised to discuss any medications they are taking with their neurologist/GP prior to conception. Table 7.4 lists some of the more common medications used which should be stopped if possible. This list is intended as an illustration only of the types of medications that may cause problems. Any woman who is taking medication should discuss this with her doctor as advice may differ for individuals, balancing the symptomatic relief gained against potential risks to the foetus and the woman herself.

Beta interferon and glatiramar acetate should be stopped about a month prior to any attempts at conception and cannot be restarted until the mother has finished breastfeeding. There have as yet been no studies done examining the effect of beta interferons on the foetus although there are concerns that they may cause miscarriage. There have been cases of women taking beta interferon who have had unplanned pregnancies and who have remained on treatment for the first few weeks of the pregnancy. Once they realised they were pregnant they stopped immediately and both later gave birth to healthy full-term babies (Burgess, unpublished data).

Table 7.4 A list of medications that should be stopped if possible during pregnancy and while breastfeeding (in consultation with a neurologist)

- Carbamazepine
- Gabapentin
- Epilim
- Interferon
- Amantadine
- Amitriptyline
- Baclofen
- Imipramine
- Methyl prednisolone (OK in moderation)

Pregnancy

Having MS does not directly affect fertility although if one partner is experiencing some sexual dysfunction, these problems may need to be addressed before the couple can conceive. Once the woman has become pregnant her MS normally goes into a period of remission although this can be offset somewhat by increased fatigue in the later stages of pregnancy. It is likely that the neurologist and/or MS specialist nurse will review the mother regularly throughout the pregnancy and continue to offer the couple support and advice.

The birth

For the vast majority of women with MS there is no special care required during the birth. Epidural anaesthetic has been shown to have no adverse effects on MS (Confavreux *et al.*, 1998) and can be used if required. Occasionally symptoms such as reduced sensation, spasms, poor mobility etc. may make practical issues difficult (e.g. getting on and off the examination couch). The nurse and interdisciplinary team can work closely with the midwives to minimise any potential problems.

Post-natal period

The weeks and months after the birth of a child are arguably the most wonderful and most stressful time of a parent's life. Intense emotional highs are followed in a matter of what seems like seconds by equally intense lows. The added complication of one partner having MS adds to the fear, fatigue and uncertainty.

The family needs practical help and support from their extended family, friends and health care professionals. It is important that the partner with MS gets a good night's sleep and as much rest as they need during the day. While helping to ease the fatigue experienced, resting may also serve to compound the guilt that many parents feel at being 'different' and not being able to do as much for their child as they want to. When things become more difficult and particularly if a relapse is experienced, doubts about whether or not having a child was the right thing to do may creep in. It is the nurse's role to reassure and support the family through this period. The doubts will settle – usually very quickly with the appropriate treatment, help and support.

Health visitors will be involved, as they are with any birth, and they need to be aware of the added problems, both physical and psychological that MS can cause. If there are other young children in the family, the health visitor may discuss with the parents the child care options available. This can ensure that the parents get time alone with the new baby and a chance to get some rest, leaving them better able to meet the needs of their older child on their return.

The neurologist and/or MS specialist nurse will endeavour to monitor the woman with MS closely during the first 12 months post-natally.

Diagnosis of MS following pregnancy

Some women experience their first troublesome relapse after the birth of their child and are diagnosed at this stage. They will need particular support and education about the disease. Occasionally mothers may blame the baby for their MS; however they should be reassured that the MS was already present, if undetected, and that the birth of their baby has merely precipitated an attack and not the disease itself.

CHAPTER 8

Cognitive dysfunction and depression in MS

Introduction

One of the first questions most people ask when first diagnosed with MS is, 'Will it affect my mind?' The answer to this question is not straightforward. Generally, what the patient really wants to know is whether or not they will acquire some type of dementia as a result of MS. This is very rarely the case, although cognitive processes such as memory, word finding, concentration and processing of information can be affected to varying degrees. Very rarely, individuals with severe MS can develop profound cognitive dysfunction.

Many people diagnosed with MS experience a variety of negative emotions. This is a very normal and necessary part of the process of adaptation. People often feel sorrow, anger, frustration or anxiety and many people feel low in mood at different times and for different reasons. Sometimes however the low mood can become more serious and may develop into depression and when this happens, the individual will need appropriate help and support.

Although Charcot recognised mood disorders in the patients he observed, it was believed for many years that MS did not affect cognitive function and to this day, problems with cognition are probably some of the least well recognised. Not everyone with MS will develop difficulties with cognitive function, for others cognitive difficulties may develop late in the disease or, on some occasions, may be the only presenting symptom. As with everything in MS, people experience varying degrees and forms of cognitive dysfunction at different stages of the disease. Understandably, these can be among some of the most distressing symptoms to be experienced for both the patient and their family. However once the problems are recognised as a symptom of MS, by the patient and their clinician, a number of strategies can be employed and the individual and their family can receive the help and advice they need.

While many cognitive problems are a direct consequence of MS, there is not always a clear demarcation between symptoms that result directly from demyelination (i.e. idiopathic) and reactive symptoms that occur as a response to the difficulties of living with MS. For example, depression may be idiopathic or reactive in origin, that is mood swings may occur as a response to circumstances or may be caused by plaques of MS within the brain. These symptoms will be explored in more detail below.

Depression in MS

One in two people with MS will experience a major depressive episode at some stage (Sadovnick *et al.*, 1996). Depression is used by different people to mean different things and it is important to clarify its meaning in this context. Many people, returning home from a bad day at work, will complain that they feel 'depressed'. However the clinical definition of depression goes far beyond feeling sad or miserable. To be diagnosed with clinical depression an individual must have experienced persistent and all pervasive feelings of sadness for at least two weeks. In addition they must also have experienced at least three other symptoms such as:

• altered sleep pattern;
• feelings of hopelessness;
• persistent thoughts of death;
• feelings of worthlessness or guilt;
• lack of energy;
• reduced ability to concentrate.

Diagnosis of clinical depression can be difficult, as most people with MS will experience periods of low mood. Fatigue will result in low energy and may cause disturbance of the individual's normal sleep pattern; cognitive problems may manifest as poor concentration and thus, what is actually a severe depressive episode may be masked or go unnoticed by others. Alternatively, someone may be diagnosed as being depressed when the symptoms they are exhibiting are actually due to the fatigue etc. resulting from their MS. It is important, however, that people with MS and their partners, as well as health care professionals, are aware of the symptoms of depression. The individual's partner often first notices these. If they are aware of the possibility of depression then appropriate help and treatment can be accessed sooner rather than later.

If someone becomes clinically depressed, treatment – usually a combination of medication and psychotherapy – is imperative. The suicide rate among people with MS has been shown to be much higher than for the general population and is one of the leading causes of death among people with MS (Sadovnick *et al.*, 1991; Koch-Herrikson and Brønnum-Hansen, 1999). Treatment can be very effective and can lead to much improved quality of life for the individual and their family.

Aetiology of depression

The reason why so many people with MS develop clinical depression is unclear. The prevalence of depression in MS is greater than for people with other neurological diseases such as Parkinson's disease. Many studies have been undertaken to try and determine the relationship of depression to a number of factors such as lesion load, disability and genetic predisposition in an attempt to understand the aetiology (Remick and Sadovnick, 1997).

Unfortunately the results of the studies have proved largely inconclusive. In practice, it is most likely that depression in MS can be caused by a number of different factors in different individuals and this should be taken into account when diagnosing and treating people (Feinstein, 1995).

Role of the nurse

One of the main barriers to treating people who have become depressed is failure to recognise the depression. The person who is feeling depressed may not have insight into the severity of their problem or may be feeling so hopeless and worthless that they become withdrawn and do not let even close family members know the extent of their feelings. Thus a potentially treatable, while very debilitating, symptom is often missed.

The chance of developing clinical depression at least once, for someone with MS is 50%. It is useful, therefore, for the nurse or health care professional, to be aware of this statistic when working with individuals with MS.

Assessment of a person with suspected depression

Sensitive but routine questioning can usually elicit the presence of depressive symptoms. If the nurse suspects an individual may be depressed or is alerted by a friend or relative of the patient, they must act. However the particular action to be taken by the nurse will vary depending upon their level of experience. Their knowledge of both MS and depression, their relationship with the patient, their feeling of ease with the situation and the time available will all have an influence on the nurse's course of action.

If the nurse feels able to talk to the patient themselves they must ensure a quiet environment which is free from interruptions. They must also ensure that both they and the patient have sufficient time to spend on what may potentially become a long and in depth session. The nurse must be prepared for the patient's reaction to talking about feelings for what may be the first time and should take care not to release thoughts or feelings within the patient that cannot be dealt with at the time. If in doubt, don't ask the questions, ask for help.

It is not unreasonable that a nurse does not feel confident in broaching the subject of depression with a patient. The nurse may also be restricted in terms of having enough time to spend with any one individual. However, every nurse should be able to ask a few simple questions to determine whether or not the individual is likely to be depressed. The nurse should then discuss their concerns with the GP/neurologist and/or MS specialist nurse. In this way the patient can be given appropriate support and treatment.

The key components of clinical depression as described below should form the basis for an initial assessment.

- How are you feeling in yourself?
- How long have you been feeling like this?
- Have you noticed any change in your sleeping pattern?
- Has your appetite changed recently?
- Are you able to enjoy the things that normally make you happy?
- Have you noted any recent loss of interest?

Questions about fatigue and concentration are usually included when making an assessment of low mood, however these symptoms are often present in MS regardless of whether or not the individual is depressed. They are not therefore, particularly useful in this context.

If an individual admits to feeling low and demonstrates most of the other features mentioned, there is a good likelihood that they are in fact depressed.

In milder forms of depression, the experienced nurse may well be able to use counselling skills and encourage the patient to discuss some of their fears and concerns. In more severe depression this will be beyond most nurses scope and the patient should be referred as a matter of urgency to a counsellor or a psychologist via their GP or neurologist. The MS specialist nurse may also be able to provide ongoing support to the person with MS and their family.

When someone with MS becomes depressed it usually affects the whole family. The person with MS is often aware of this, which compounds their feelings of guilt and worthlessness, i.e. of 'being a burden'. By supporting the family and teaching them about depression and the available treatments, the nurse can help to relieve some of their fears and anxieties.

Role of the doctor

In the same way as described above, the doctor should always be aware that there is quite a high likelihood of depression among people with MS. If they feel an individual is particularly low in mood, routine questioning such as that described above should be made to establish the likelihood of an individual suffering from depression. If depression is suspected, the doctor should also try and evaluate the risk of suicide. As previously mentioned, suicide rates among people with MS are much higher than for the general population. Risk factors for suicide are listed in Table 8.1. Individuals thought to exhibit a moderate to severe risk of suicide by the doctor, should be considered as requiring immediate follow up with a possible need for hospitalisation.

The doctor should also initiate a treatment regime. This may be anti-depressant medication or referral to a counsellor or psychologist (often, a combination of medication and counselling/psychotherapy is used to

Table 8.1 Risk factors for suicide

- Single male (particularly if widowed or divorced)[1]
- Unemployment[1]
- Family history of suicide[1]
- Alcohol or drug abuse[1]
- Previous suicide attempt[2]
- Lack of social support[2]
- Onset of MS within the last 5 years and subsequent development of moderate-severe disability[3]

1. Remick and Sadovnick, 1997
2. Ebers and Paty, 1998
3. Weinshenker, 1997

good effect). There are few specific guidelines relating to the treatment of depression in MS and everyone should be treated individually depending on their particular circumstances. Studies have shown that a combination of anti-depressants and counselling can be effective (Feinstein, 2000).

There are two main types of anti-depressants in common use: tricyclic anti-depressants such as amitriptyline and imipramine and the newer selective serotonin reuptake inhibitors (SSRIs). There is no particular anti-depressant that has been shown to be more effective in MS than others. The choice of medication should be made on an individual basis.

The side effects of the tricyclic anti-depressants tend to be more pronounced than those of the SSRIs. Symptoms such as dizziness, dry mouth and constipation may mean that patients are more likely to discontinue treatment or can only tolerate sub-therapeutic doses (Schiffer and Wineman, 1990).

The SSRIs (which include fluoxetine, paroxetine, sertraline, fluvox-amine and citalopram) are no more effective than the tricyclic anti-depressants but tend to be better tolerated. One of the main side effects experienced is impairment of sexual function. It is known that libido and sexual performance are impaired in at least 20% of healthy individuals taking SSRIs (Walker et al., 1993). As many people with MS already experience some degree of sexual dysfunction, alternative treatments may need to be considered such as counselling or psychotherapy.

The pros and cons of the different anti-depressants available should be discussed with the individual in the context of their particular needs.

Counselling

This is a very useful therapy in the treatment of depression and other mood disorders. Counselling alone may be sufficient to lift an individual's mood in mild–moderate depression or it may be used in conjunction with anti-depressants. People with moderate–severe depression may well need the more structured input of a psychologist or psychiatrist.

Any form of counselling should be approached with flexibility and an open mind. MS is such a variable disease, each individual experiences relapses and remissions and faces an uncertain future. The physical symptoms of their MS at any given time will of course impact on the patient's mood. Thus any form of counselling, whether it be support from nursing staff or insight-based therapy from a trained counsellor should be flexible enough and of sufficient duration to meet the individual's needs which may change over time (Minden, 1992).

Mood swings

Many people with MS experience frequent mood swings. Often it is their families that first recognise this is happening. These are usually just a normal response to the uncertainties, frustrations and fatigue that MS brings. It is often simple things that trigger a mood swing such as dropping a cup, trying to fasten a button or cut up a meal. The fatigue that is so often a feature of MS also tends to make people more short-tempered. With support and understanding the person with MS and their family can learn to manage mood swings more effectively.

For others, the MS itself can cause some emotional lability. People may find themselves crying at things that would not normally have affected them such as a sad film (or even a happy film) or a mild rebuke from their partner. This sort of tearfulness is separate from that which results from depression. Both the person with MS and their partner may find the frequent crying difficult to understand. As nurses we can explain that this is part of the MS in the same way that pins and needles or fatigue can be. Once the family understands this, they are able to develop appropriate coping strategies. The person with MS may be able to identify triggers, such as those mentioned above, and either avoid them or prepare themselves and others. Often an unobtrusive relaxation exercise such as deep breathing or focusing on relaxing one particular part of their body (e.g. shoulders) can be helpful. Each individual will devise their own coping methods once they understand why they are behaving in this way.

This type of uncontrollable laughing or crying affects about 10% of people with MS. This phenomenon (known variously as 'emotional release', 'emotional incontinence' and 'pathological laughing and crying') has an unclear aetiology. It is thought that the cortex, bulbar nuclei and the hypothalamus all play a part. There is also speculation that the different hemispheres of the brain have a different emphasis. For example, pathological laughter seems to be largely right sided while crying is associated with left-sided (or dominant hemisphere) lesions. However it is rarely as simple as this. It is likely that gender also plays a role; more women suffer from pathological crying while more men experience pathological laughter (Feinstein, 1999). The aetiology of this phenomenon is likely to be a combination of many different factors.

Treatment involves a two-pronged approach. Firstly, as with everything in MS, it is important that both the person with MS and their family, friends and colleagues understand why they behave in this way. This helps to prevent others from losing patience with the individual or feeling hurt when they apparently respond inappropriately to a confidence etc.

Medication can also be very helpful in controlling these episodes. Amitriptyline in doses of up to 75mg daily has been shown to be very effective with an improvement noted within 48 hours (well before any anti-depressant effect would be noted) (Schiffer *et al.*, 1985).

Case study 4

BG is a 28-year-old man who is in a stable relationship with his partner. He works full time as an accountant. BG attended the clinic and was obviously distressed by some problem. On closer questioning by the MS specialist nurse and neurologist, BG admitted that he had recently started to burst into laughter during meetings at work and on one occasion over a romantic dinner with his partner. He did not understand why he had started laughing and did not associate it with his MS. Both his colleagues and his partner were unsure what to make of his recent behaviour. BG admitted he thought he was 'going mad'. The MS nurse explained the aetiology of pathological laughing to BG and the neurologist prescribed 50mg amitriptyline nightly. BG felt happier just knowing that he was not 'going mad'. He was able to share this information with his partner and manager at work. The MS nurse contacted him by phone a week later to assess the effectiveness of the amitriptyline. BG reported that he was feeling much better and reported no further outbursts over the preceding four days. He continued to do well on the amitriptyline.

Euphoria

Sometimes people with MS become euphoric, i.e. happy with their circumstances, irrespective of their disability and other problems. They often appear to have little insight into their difficulties. This euphoric state of mind is fixed and rarely varies. Again the pathology causing euphoria is unclear, although studies have shown that it tends to be linked with the extensive cerebral damage often seen in advanced MS (Rabins *et al.*, 1986; Ron and Logsdail, 1989).

Treatment for euphoria is not usually pursued. In practice it makes coping with the problems of MS much easier for the individual themselves, their family and also health care professionals working with them.

Case study 5

AM was 42 years old, married with no children. She had been diagnosed with MS 20 years previously and was severely disabled. She was unable to meet any of her personal care needs and was largely confined to bed. She was admitted to the neurology ward for assessment of swallowing problems. Before treatment of her swallowing problems could proceed, AM developed pneumonia and became very ill. Her MS worsened during this episode. However throughout her stay and the acute episodes, AM remained happy and cheerful, she was always grateful for any care given her and was always glad to see her husband and family. This made coping with a very difficult period much more bearable for all concerned. AM's partner gained a lot of comfort from knowing that she was cushioned somewhat from the reality of the disease by the euphoria.

Cognitive dysfunction

Many people with MS, at all levels of disability, often remark that their memory has got worse or that they have problems following the plot of a book or film. These are typical symptoms of the type of cognitive impairment often seen in MS.

Cognition can be loosely defined as the processes involved in memory, reasoning, attention, concentration and visuospatial perception. A study of people with MS that concentrated on these particular aspects of cognition, found that the frequency of cognitive impairment was 43% (Rao *et al.*, 1991).

In practice cognitive impairment varies from barely noticeable problems with short-term memory or word finding to quite severe difficulties with memory and concentration, often combined with poor insight into these difficulties. Fortunately severe cognitive deficits are rare. In the same way as other impairments experienced by the person with MS, each person will follow a unique course. Cognitive problems may also come and go over time, as many other symptoms of MS may do (Langdon, 1997).

Diagnosing cognitive impairment

For most people with MS, who have only mild and often fluctuating cognitive impairment, their problems are rarely evident to others outside the immediate family. It is usually difficult for health care professionals working with them to detect any deficits. Doctors routinely use the mini mental state test (MMS) when assessing cognitive impairment in patients. This test asks questions such as: What year is it? Who is the Prime Minister? What is the date? etc.; and will detect only severe cognitive dysfunction. It is usually the person with MS or their close family that will remark to the doctor or nurse that their 'memory is shot' or that they keep forgetting the plot of the book they are reading. This is the cue for a more in depth assessment of the problems faced by the individual.

The nature of the dysfunction is best assessed by psychologists who have a battery of assessments at their fingertips. This can take several hours and indeed two to three days on occasions. Psychological testing only tends to be used therefore, if the impairments are causing the individual moderate to severe problems in their day-to-day lives. It usually falls to the MS specialist nurse to assess the impact of the cognitive impairments reported by the patient and/or their partner on their lives, and liaise accordingly with the appropriate member of the interdisciplinary team.

Memory loss

Memory loss is one of the most common types of cognitive dysfunction experienced by people with MS. It can manifest as mildly irritating, as in the following example:

> I have to write down all my appointments etc. in my diary or I forget them, and I'm forever going into the kitchen for something and forgetting what I wanted.
> (LM – 28 years old, single, works in a record shop)

Or it may become severely disabling as illustrated in this example:

> I can no longer even follow the thread of a conversation. We met up with some old friends last week and started talking about old times. I couldn't remember any of it. You could see they were wondering what was happening. I even forget the boys' birthdays – things like that all fall to my husband now.
> (SW – 46 years old, married with two boys, 18 and 16)

Memory problems are often not perceived as being connected with MS. People attribute their failing memory to old age or stress, or may worry that something more sinister is happening to them. By discussing the potential problems with people with MS and their families, much of the anxiety, frustration, and misunderstandings that frequently occur can be prevented.

There are many different strategies that can be employed to compensate for memory problems depending on the particular difficulties experienced. Often an occupational therapist can work with an individual and help them to evolve coping strategies. For example, if someone is having problems remembering which tablets to take, obtaining a dosette box from the chemist may be helpful. People often forget appointments etc. and if they can get into a routine of writing anything they need to remember in a diary or notebook, and remember to check it daily, much of this can be alleviated. The psychologist can also be very helpful if the individual has more severe problems. They can work with the individual to devise appropriate coping strategies. Understanding, help and support from family members is invaluable.

Problem solving

Solving problems or making decisions can be difficult for people with MS if their reasoning and judgement is impaired. Impairment of reasoning is difficult to detect and tends to be demonstrated through poor decisions being made as a result of faulty reasoning, for example:

> I saw a Christmas card for my husband on the market which was just what I wanted. I was just going to get it when I saw my husband returning from the car park. I thought he might see the card although he was still some distance away so I replaced it on the stall. It was only when we got home that I realised I should have bought it. I made my husband drive all the way back to market so that I could buy it.
>
> (AF – 60 years old, married and has had MS for five years)

In this example AF decides not to buy the card initially as she reasons that her husband will see the card even though he is a considerable distance away. Having decided not to buy the card, AF then realises that her reasoning was at fault, but rather than going to the local shop for a card, she asks her husband to drive several miles back to the market so that she could buy the original card.

Again there is no specific treatment for these sorts of problems. It is largely a case of understanding and accepting the limitations imposed by these deficits. These problems can be difficult to accept and the person with MS and their family will need a lot of support and understanding throughout this process. The nurse is often the individual providing this support, be it on a ward, in the community or as an MS specialist nurse. The nurse too should ensure that they receive appropriate support from colleagues as required.

Attention and concentration

An individual's ability to pay attention or concentrate on more than one thing at a time may become impaired. We are frequently required to attend to two or more things at the same time, for example, driving the car while listening to our children talking about their day at school or perhaps using the computer while talking to a customer on the telephone. These multiple tasks can become very difficult for some people with MS to manage, they become distracted and are often unable to exclude irrelevant stimuli from their surroundings which impinge on their consciousness. This can make them much slower or unable to fulfil two or more tasks simultaneously.

In order to overcome these particular problems, the person with MS first needs to understand the difficulties they are having and that they are a symptom of the MS. They can then share this with their family and colleagues as and when they feel it is appropriate.

Once the problem is understood the patient can then be helped to develop coping strategies. This may be the role of the psychologist, occupational therapist, MS nurse or other member of the interdisciplinary team depending on the nature of the problems experienced. Whichever health care professional works with the patient it is important that the individual's context both at home and at work is understood. Only by appreciating the full picture can coping strategies that work be evolved.

Case study 6

LP is a full-time mother. She has had MS for five years and other than fatigue and some sensory symptoms, she manages quite well. She has two children, M who is seven years old and B who is eight years old; both attend the local junior school. LP drives the mile to school each afternoon to pick the children up (she finds this too far to walk easily). Both children enjoy school and naturally want to tell LP about their day. LP contacted her specialist nurse to say that she was becoming concerned that she was, 'taking things out' on the children.

LP was seen in clinic and she and the MS nurse discussed the problems. It became clear that LP was only short-tempered with the children when she had another task she needed to concentrate on. This had come to a head over the last month when picking the children up from school she had found she could not concentrate on both her driving and the children talking. The MS nurse spent some time with LP explaining the problems some people experience with attention and concentration.

Once LP understood why she was finding it difficult to give her children the attention they needed at times, she was able to compensate for this.

She explained to her children that, 'mummy could not listen to them talking and concentrate on her driving at the same time', but stressed that she did want to know about their day. She set aside some time after picking the children up for them to tell her about their most pressing news and then the children were quiet for the ten-minute drive back home. This worked well and LP was able to apply similar strategies to other pressure points through the day.

Summary

Approximately half of all people with MS will experience depression at some stage during their life. This often goes undetected and nurses and other health care professionals should always be alert to the possibility when working with an individual. Simple questioning can usually be sufficient to determine whether or not someone is depressed. The individual should then be seen by their doctor and/or a counsellor or psychologist. It is known that anti-depressants either alone or in combination with counselling can be very effective.

Other cognitive problems tend to be mild for the majority of people with MS. Problems with memory, word finding, reasoning and attention may be experienced. A small number of individuals (approximately 5–10%) will have more severe cognitive problems making it difficult for them to maintain their roles both at home and at work.

As with other symptoms of MS, cognitive problems can come and go over time. Other symptoms, such as fatigue, will also impact on any cognitive problems.

Individuals and families experiencing these types of difficulties often need a great deal of support to work through cognitive problems. The nurse should ensure that the individual understands their problems are related to MS and should liaise with the appropriate member of the interdisciplinary team (i.e. GP, neurologist, psychologist, MS specialist nurse or occupational therapist). Compensatory strategies relevant to the individual can then be developed.

CHAPTER 9

Patient-centred nursing in MS

Introduction

As has been demonstrated in previous chapters, the needs of someone with MS are usually multi-layered and complex. No one symptom can be viewed in isolation as each will impact on the individual in many different ways. MS has an influence on every sphere of an individual's life, affecting them physically, emotionally, socially and financially. It affects their ability to work, their role within the family, the life choices open to them and of course touches their whole family in different but equally significant ways. Because MS is all pervasive and affects every aspect of an individual's life, nursing someone with MS necessitates a holistic approach to providing individualised patient care and requires the nurse to fulfil many different roles.

Virginia Henderson who was born in America in 1897 spent her life nursing and writing about nursing. Her definition of nursing is still relevant today. She writes:

> I believe that the function the nurse performs is primarily an independent one – that of acting for the patient when he lacks knowledge, physical strength, or the will to act for himself as he would ordinarily act in health, or in carrying out prescribed therapy. This function is seen as complex and creative, as offering unlimited opportunity for the application of the physical, biological and social sciences and the development of the skills based on them (Henderson, 1966).

This definition was written in the 1960s and continues to form the bedrock of much of nursing today; however, the role of the nurse is now much more far-reaching. Holistic, patient-centred care requires that the emphasis of care shifts from nurses doing things to and for patients to the patient themselves becoming an active partner in their care. The role of the nurse is to empower the patient to deal with the problems they are facing (Binnie and Titchen, 1999). Thus the interaction between nurse and patient becomes part of a dynamic exchange and underpins a therapeutic nurse–patient relationship.

Patient-centred care requires the nurse to see the experience of MS through the patient's eyes. The nurse must be able to demonstrate empathy and develop a rapport with the individual. In this way the patient is shown that the nurse values the person inside the patient and does not see them as just someone else with MS (Hawksey and Williams, 2000). The individual, their priorities and needs must become the focus of care.

In order to achieve patient-centred nursing continuity of care is essential. If the patient is being cared for by a succession of different nurses, it is almost impossible for a nurse to develop the understanding and empathy with a particular patient that is essential to providing patient-centred care. Team nursing, which is widely practised, moves some way towards this although responsibility for decisions regarding care tends to vary from shift to shift. Primary nursing where one nurse has responsibility for the nursing management of a given patient, leaving directions for their care in their absence, comes much closer to the ideal. Indeed primary nursing has been described as 'a view of nursing as professional, patient-centred practice' (Hegevary, 1982).

It is recognised that practising true primary care and developing patient-centred practice is often very difficult and there can be many obstacles along the way. Many nurses find change difficult and implementing change can be even harder. The NHS can be likened to a very large ship; it takes a long, long time to change direction. However it is very important that as nurses we strive towards this type of nursing, particularly when working with people with MS. The needs of people with MS and their families are so varied, changing and ongoing that they can only truly be met as we move towards patient-centred nursing and an understanding of the benefits to both patient and nurse from a therapeutic nurse–patient relationship.

The different roles a nurse will be required to fulfil in providing comprehensive and holistic care for people with MS and their families and in developing an effective nurse–patient relationship are listed in Figure 9.1. Each of these roles is important and will be explored below.

Assessment

The assessment process is key. If done properly, it will form the basis for all future care of the individual. As well as being the best opportunity for

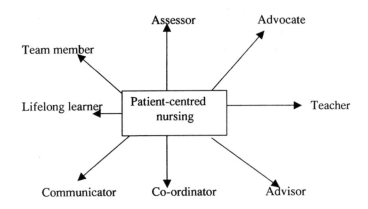

Figure 9.1 Some of the different roles a nurse must fulfil when working with people with MS.

establishing the patient's needs and problems it can lay the foundations for the development of an effective nurse–patient relationship. This relationship may stretch across many years as patients often return to the same health care team many times as their needs change. Assessment should also be an ongoing and integral theme within the patient's care plan as part of the nursing process. MS is characterised by unpredictability and change, and so the individual's needs constantly change over time and should be reassessed as required.

There are a number of factors to consider before commencing an assessment. The nurse needs a basic understanding of MS, its impact and the available treatment options. It is more than likely that the patient will have questions of their own that they wish to ask the nurse. The nurse should be prepared for this and have at least some of the answers to hand. It is also useful to have some information leaflets and some contact numbers (e.g. the MS specialist nurse and/or MS Society) available if appropriate.

It is important that the nurse should take time before meeting the patient to review their medical notes and other team members' notes if available. The needs of someone who is newly diagnosed are likely to be very different to those of someone who has had MS for many years. It is also necessary to understand something of the context of the patient before the assessment. For example, are they employed? have they any children? what is their marital status? do they have anyone else in the family with MS? This latter factor in particular may result in unfounded fears and concerns which often affect the way the individual approaches their own MS. If the nurse is aware of this potential, they can explore the patient's prior experience with them and go some way towards providing appropriate reassurance. By studying the patient's notes prior to the assessment it is ensured that the nurse approaches the meeting with some appreciation of potentially sensitive areas and is able to proceed with tact and empathy.

In an ideal world, the assessment would take place in a quiet area free from interruptions. This is often not possible but privacy should be considered at all times – patients are more likely to discuss sensitive issues with the nurse somewhere they feel comfortable and safe, rather than with no more than a curtain separating them from the rest of the ward.

Nurses who have the opportunity will find it helpful to visit the patient at home on at least one occasion. Community nurses are able to exploit these advantages to the full. Seeing the patient at home gives the nurse an invaluable opportunity to assess not only the individual but also their accommodation, access into and around their home etc. The nurse may also meet other family members who they would not otherwise see. In this way, it is often possible to gain a general impression as to how well the patient and their family are coping with the problems facing them. It is very difficult to practise in a truly holistic way in hospital, the patient becomes just that – a patient and becomes separated from their normal context. Visiting people at home ensures that the individual is much more comfortable and has his or her sense of self intact – you are their guest rather than vice versa. As a result people are often more open in any discussion of their needs, allowing a fuller picture of the impact of MS on them and their family to be gained.

The structure of the assessment interview is likely to be governed to a large extent by whichever model of nursing is being used. This may be based on the activities of daily living as described by Roper *et al.* (1996) or the self-care deficit model described by Orem (1990) or one of the many other nursing models that abound within nursing literature. However the nurse must ensure that each assessment is tailored to the individual and that they do not merely recite the same formula with each patient. A model of nursing should act as a framework or philosophy underpinning patient care and should not be viewed as a recipe to be followed no matter what. In the real world both patients and nurses experience real problems that require insight, resourcefulness, empathy and good communication to solve (Walsh, 1998). The concept of patient-centred care should be uppermost when making a patient assessment.

When assessing people with MS, the nurse should not merely rely on questions and answers but should also be alert for any non-verbal cues.

For example, the nurse may notice that the patient appears very dry when talking. This can be a sign that the person with MS has cut back on fluids because of bladder problems or that they are experiencing side effects from anti-cholinergic medication. Another example is patients with more advanced disease who sit with their arms tightly folded, this can sometimes be because of a tremor. Does the patient have any cuts or bruises – this may be an indication that they are falling. Watch the individual walking – how steady are they?; does their gait appear normal? All these and more can provide the nurse with indications of potential symptoms and the nurse should direct their questions appropriately.

Once a problem or need is identified, closer questioning and discussion with the patient can help to determine the exact nature of the problem and its impact. Examples of the sort of questions to ask when a particular problem is identified are contained within the relevant chapters.

Throughout the interview the nurse will need to use a number of different skills. Communication skills are central and this involves listening as well as questioning. People with MS, particularly those who have lived with it for some time, are often very knowledgeable. This can sometimes feel threatening to the health care professional, particularly if they are themselves inexperienced in this area, however this should be viewed more as an opportunity and a resource than a threat. Sharing knowledge in this way can reinforce feelings of mutual respect which is one of the corner stones of a therapeutic nurse–patient relationship and learning from each other can provide a solid foundation on which to build and develop.

Throughout the assessment the nurse should try to ascertain what the patient's priorities are. All too often the patient's own concerns get overlooked. It has been shown that patients tend to be more concerned with problems such as fatigue and cognition while health care professionals (particularly clinicians) tend to focus on people's physical disabilities (Rothwell *et al.*, 1997). A more recent study of almost 900 health professionals and people with MS highlighted many differences in the focus of managing MS. The study also showed that there are many shared views and that in some cases people with MS are more realistic about their disease than clinicians (Bates *et al.*, 1999). This emphasises the need to ensure that it is the patient's priorities that are central to any plan of care and that the patient is fully included in any decision-making etc. Our aim is to enable patients to fulfil their own goals and needs.

Once the nurse is able to ascertain the patient's priorities and needs, the nurse should then communicate these needs to the rest of the team.

As the patient realises that the nurse has placed their priorities at the centre of the plan of care and is demonstrating empathy, so patient-centred nursing becomes more of a reality.

The development of a therapeutic nurse–patient relationship takes time. One model that has been used to describe its development is Peplau's interpersonal relations model (McGuinness and Peters, 1999). This describes the process as a series of overlapping stages. While this may sound complex, its essence is relatively simple and the model is used to describe the way in which a collaborative relationship can develop between nurse and patient. This is essential in allowing effective problem-solving that has real meaning to the patient and in establishing a relationship that may stretch across many years.

The four stages described by the model are orientation, identification, exploitation and resolution. Peplau's model has been used largely within the field of mental health nursing but it is gradually becoming more widely used within general nursing.

Orientation is the phase at which the nurse–patient relationship begins – the patient has a need and seeks assistance. The nurse and patient begin to work together to identify and prioritise needs and to establish why help is required. Seeing the problems as part of life and as an opportunity for learning can help the individual to grow and develop and can be used to turn the experience into a positive event (Walsh, 1998).

Identification describes the strengthening of the nurse–patient relationship. The patient begins to gain confidence in discussing their fears and concerns with the nurse. The nurse's role becomes that of advisor and teacher during this phase.

The exploitation phase is that in which the patient and their family begin to take control. They begin to search actively for information and answers to their problems. During this phase the nurse needs to act as both a resource and as an advisor.

The resolution phase is that at which the patient becomes independent of the nurse and the nurse–patient relationship is dissolved. This is not a realistic end-point in MS due to the progressive and unpredictable nature of the disease. However, an episode of care may come to a conclusion (for example, an inpatient stay or specific treatment such as a wound dressing). It is likely, however, that the patient will return to the health care team in the future and the nurse–patient relationship can be continued.

It is not suggested that nurses should follow this model to the exclusion of others. However, it may prove a useful adjunct to their existing model of nursing and may provide some structure when considering patient-centred nursing.

Having completed an assessment, the nurse must then decide how best to proceed with the information gained. The most thorough and empathetic assessment is useless if the insights gained are not followed through and communicated to the rest of the team. The importance of thorough and appropriate documentation must not be overlooked.

Team member/co-ordinator

The nurse does not work alone but as a member of a team of health and social care professionals. The immediate team may be small, perhaps only a nurse and general practitioner, but there will be other team members that can be called on as required and each team member has a specific role to play in meeting the patient's needs. When the team is working together effectively, the whole will be greater then the sum of its individual parts. The team cannot work effectively without good communication and liaison between members.

Once a nurse has completed a patient assessment, the information and insights gained as well as the patient's concerns and priorities should be shared with the team. A co-ordinated plan of care should then be decided upon in full consultation with the patient. It is essential that the patient and their family are involved in and remain central to this plan of care.

> Providing accurate and timely information is crucial to rehabilitation care. The nurse will have knowledge of each disciplines rehabilitative therapeutic interventions as well as a comprehensive understanding of the process of rehabilitation. This allows discussion of the team's approach with the patient and the patient's family (Hawksey and Williams, 2000).

Thus the nurse's role as co-ordinator, communicator and advocate is required to be ongoing for the duration of his or her involvement with the patient and their family.

It is worth at this point discussing rehabilitation as a concept. There are many different definitions of rehabilitation, for example:

> A process of active change by which a person, who has become disabled, acquires the knowledge and skills needed for optimal physical, psychological and social function (Compston et al., 1993).

> A process aiming to restore personal autonomy in those aspects of daily living considered most relevant by patients or service users and their family carers (Sinclair and Dickinson, 1998).

All these definitions are concerned with helping the individual to gain as much independence and function as they are able to in all spheres of their life. This philosophy is also at the core of patient-centred nursing and rehabilitation as a term is interchangeable with this. Thus, throughout this book, discussion about the role of the nurse in caring for people with MS is synonymous with rehabilitation.

Rehabilitation should not be viewed as a separate 'therapy' that takes place only in specialised units, but as the care that someone with MS requires and should receive throughout their lifetime from all members of the interdisciplinary team.

Advocacy

The nurse's role as patient advocate is particularly important when practising holistic, patient-centred care. The Collins English Dictionary defines an advocate variously as someone who supports or recommends a course of action publicly; someone who upholds or defends a cause and as a person who intercedes on behalf of another (1990). A nurse is often required to fulfil all these definitions of advocacy when working with people with MS and their families.

The role of advocate can be applied at different levels:

- immediate sphere of practice (e.g. ward);
- directorate or health centre;
- hospital trust or primary care group;
- local health authority/ board or primary care trust;
- regional health authority/ board;
- governmental level.

Not every nurse by any means, will wish to or feel able to act as an advocate at all these levels; however, every nurse should be aware of the different spheres of influence they can affect.

Working as an effective advocate, at whatever level, comes back to good communication skills and patient-centred nursing. The nurse must be sure that they are working with the patient when acting as their advocate and are not operating independently of the patient because they feel 'they know best'. As has been noted previously, the patient's priorities and concerns may well be different from those of the team working with them and it is the role of the nurse to work with the patient in communicating these priorities to the rest of the team.

Advocacy is not only putting the patient's views to the interdisciplinary team, but also explaining the rationale behind proposed treatments and care packages to the patient and their family. Once the patient understands the options available to them and why the team want to work with them in a particular way, the patient is in a position to make informed choices about the suggested package of care. The nurse should also ensure that the patient is aware of their rights regarding benefits (e.g. disability living allowance), employment etc., the nurse may well need to refer the patient to a social worker for any detailed discussions. The patient should also be made aware of resources such as the MS Society which can provide help and support both locally and nationally.

Facts are the tools of advocacy (Price, 1997) and the nurse should take every opportunity to learn – be it understanding MS, its management and impact on people with MS or finding out about local and national resources. For nurses who feel that they want to, or are able to get involved in advocacy at a higher level, a working knowledge of the way in which policies are written, and of who should be approached on which committee to ensure that MS is on the agenda, is always invaluable. The line manager or GP/consultant can often be very helpful in this respect. If working at higher levels, the Royal College of Nursing (RCN) can also be invaluable in providing advice and support to nurses trying to improve conditions for people with MS. For example the RCN, in conjunction with MS specialist nurses, put forward submissions and a subsequent appeal to the National Institute for Clinical Excellence (NICE) regarding the guidance they had issued advising that interferons should not be prescribed. As a result of the appeal (in which a number of other groups including the Association of British Neurologists and the MS Society were represented) a further audit has been commissioned and the advice to doctors not to prescribe interferons has been lifted, for the time being at least (Scott, 2000). Individuals can make a difference.

Advocacy at a national level is not something that the majority of nurses are either able to or wish to be involved in. However, every nurse should understand the concept of advocacy and its importance at any level. Ensuring that an individual who experiences severe fatigue gets enough rest between tests and therapies is just as important as presenting an appeal to NICE. The patient's right to dignity, independence and informed choice should be a priority.

Teaching

Teaching forms part of the role of any nurse, no matter where they are based. Teaching in the context of MS is essential. Although many aspects of MS are unclear, it is a lifelong disease and patients must be encouraged to manage their own disease and to know when and who to ask for help. Equally the nurse is responsible for their own self-development and for increasing their own knowledge of MS, its impact and management.

A number of skills are required to teach someone – communication, collaboration, assessment of need etc. as well as an understanding of the basic principles of learning and teaching. For the most part, teaching will involve nothing more than advising patients informally about MS generally and talking to them about self-help strategies they can employ to allow them to manage their own disease more effectively.

Patients will also need to evolve positive coping strategies to help them live their life with MS. One of the mainstays of coping is hope. There are various strategies that can be used to engender hope within an individual and the nurse may well need to spend time with someone helping them to develop some appropriate strategies. Hope as a concept is discussed in more depth below.

Occasionally, nurses may be called on to teach to a larger group, for example a patient support group or a teaching session for colleagues within the interdisciplinary team. The principles remain the same – good preparation and effective communication of the points you wish to convey. Many units have regular teaching sessions where different members of the team take it in turns to teach each other about different aspects of care relative to the focus of the unit. These can be invaluable, both for gaining experience in teaching others within a safe environment and also for learning what others teach.

There are many resources available to you (and to patients) when trying to find out about a particular aspect of MS (Appendix I contains relevant addresses and websites), for example:

- other team members;
- books and journals;
- MS Society;
- MS Research Trust;
- Internet;
- conferences/study days;
- networking;
- pharmaceutical companies.

Part of teaching is learning and as developments both within MS and within nursing continue apace, the nurse needs to become a lifelong learner. The concept of lifelong learning has come much more to the fore since PREP (UKCC, 1997) was instituted. Lifelong learning is the continuing development of knowledge, competence and understanding by the individual nurse and requires the nurse to assess their own needs and set their own goals (Gopee, 2000). Because our understanding of MS, its impact and management are constantly changing, the nurse's role as lifelong learner is essential. By continually updating our understanding, our practice can be changed accordingly and the benefits passed on to people with MS as we work with them.

Hope

Hope is a word that is familiar to us all – we hope we will get the off duty we requested next weekend. Hope is not only a 'wishing for' but has a wider concept that it is important to consider when nursing people with MS. Our patients also hope for things, be this a cure, or something simple such as hoping they will feel a bit better tomorrow. Hope should be seen as a present which is full of possibilities and not of a future that may never happen. It is the courage to realise some of the hoped for possibilities that can be found by both nurse and patient within a therapeutic nurse–patient relationship (Castledine, 2000).

Despite knowing that MS is incurable, people with MS often express a great deal of hope. Hope is a sustaining force, an expression of optimism and of having a future, it underpins 'positive thinking'. This is not to say that someone with MS will be or indeed should always be optimistic and hopeful. Indeed very often they will feel low in mood and it is essential that individuals are able to grieve the losses they experience as a result of their MS. Strategies such as denial, that may initially appear counter-productive, may also be used as a positive coping strategy. Denial can allow the patient time to adapt and refocus the hopes that they have (Wilkinson, 1996).

The opposite of hope is hopelessness and an individual 'moves from hope to hopelessness from moment to moment, recognition of this ever changing process can inspire hope even in moments of despair' (Morgante, 1997).

It often falls to the nurse to assess an individual's level of hopefulness and to discuss with them strategies that can be used to feel more positive about their life and the future, more hopeful.

People who are feeling hopeless are usually depressed and the two are closely intertwined. Likewise feeling hopeful is associated with feeling positive and generally happier about circumstances. An individual's personality has a huge influence on how hopeful or otherwise they are able to remain despite problems that they face. Coping abilities, morale and sense of self all influence the way an individual feels. The individual's support network and the caring relationships they develop both with significant others and, in a different sense, with health care professionals will all have a positive impact (Forbes, 1994). Table 9.1 lists some of the resources and strategies that people can employ to encourage a feeling of hope. Not all strategies will be helpful for all individuals and the list is intended to give nurses some ideas only of the sort of strategies that can be shared with patients in an attempt to engender hope. The nurse should aim to work with people with MS and their families to help them use some of these strategies or to find some of their own in order to give the individual a sense of purpose and of self (Foote *et al.*, 1990).

In this way hope becomes an important coping strategy for all concerned. 'Hope is a fundamental aspect of human life, closely related to coping and adaptation. It can allow an individual to change from merely functioning to living as fully as possible' (Bain, 1996).

The strategies listed in Table 9.1 should not only be used to focus patients and their families but also to help the nurse cope with the often difficult and emotionally draining work of caring for people with MS.

Table 9.1 Strategies that can be used to promote hopefulness

- **Having a sense of purpose**
  Continue to work
  Attend further education classes
  Commence voluntary work
  Seeking information, self-directed learning
- **Spiritual belief**
  Finding pleasure in small things
  Having a sense of self-worth
- **Supportive and loving relationships with family and friends**
  Discuss fears and concerns with family/nurse/counsellor
  Uplifting memories
  Humour
  Having something to look forward to
- **Effective symptom management**
  Relaxation and exercise
  Improvements in environment
  Healthy diet
  Therapeutic relationship with health care team
- **Knowing your own limitations and working round them**
  Setting attainable aims

Evidence-based practice

Clinical governance has become all important within the NHS since 1999. The Department of Health published a white paper entitled 'A First Class Service' (DoH, 1999) from which the principles of clinical governance are drawn. The main principle is safe, effective, patient-centred care that is constantly developing and improving. One of the keys to providing this type of care is evidence-based practice.

Evidence-based practice is about continually questioning our practice – why are we doing it at all? is there a better way of doing it? what is the rationale for doing it this way? (Walsh and Ford, 1989). Nurses often link evidence-based practice with research and 'research' seems to have threatening connotations for a lot of nurses.

Research can mean many things and does not necessarily require the nurse to undertake their own research project (although a simple and well thought out research project should not be dismissed). Simply reading peer reviewed journals with a critical eye can be both helpful and informative. The nurse must learn to recognise scientifically sound papers from those whose methodology is not robust. There is a wealth of information available about MS and, used selectively, this can inform practice and educate nurses and so in turn, people with MS and their families.

Should a nurse or interdisciplinary team alter their practice, perhaps as a result of reading about new developments in a particular field, e.g. wound care; then the new practice needs to be evaluated and audit is invaluable for this purpose. Audits are essential for evaluating any practice – be it a new development or an existing procedure. Used properly, the results of audits can themselves be used to facilitate the change process.

Audits should be kept simple and are used to determine the effectiveness of a plan of care or treatment regime by measuring specific outcomes. Used in this way, audit can provide a rationale for practice or an agent for change, depending on the results obtained. It should be remembered that the audit process is cyclical:

Audit and research can be vital tools in a nurse's armoury, enabling care of people with MS to be continually improved and developed. The nurse working as teacher can disseminate the information gained to both staff and patients. This all leads back to the importance of assessment and patient-centred nursing.

CHAPTER 10

Health promotion and self-management for people with MS

Introduction

MS is an incurable disease and as such people with MS spend their whole lives living with the knowledge that they have MS. The strategies that people develop to help them cope with this knowledge will vary widely. The success of the different strategies employed will depend on the individual's personality, support network and attitude. As nurses we need to be able to help people with MS develop appropriate coping strategies. This includes helping people to manage their own disease so that input from health professionals is kept to a minimum and the individual is able to continue to live their life as normally as possible. Thus the nurse, in conjunction with the interdisciplinary team, should be striving to ensure that the locus of control is returned to the individual with MS.

People with MS should be actively discouraged from perceiving of themselves as 'ill'. The Wellness model (Clark, 1986), describes wellness as 'a positive striving that is unique to the individual, in which a person can be ill and still have wellness with a deep appreciation for the joy of living and with a life purpose'.

No matter what level of disability an individual is living with, many opportunities still exist for them. Activities may take rather more planning and organisation but with the right attitude and a resourceful, problem solving approach, most things can be accomplished. For example:

SJ has always enjoyed fishing. Despite now being wheelchair bound, he is still able to go fishing in certain sites, with help from his friend. When the situation is right, he will even sit in his wheelchair in the river to ensure he catches the best fish.

It is the belief that 'I can' that must be fostered rather than the belief that with the diagnosis of MS, life stops.

Nurses must help the individual to realise that they do still have a lot of potential and that with understanding, self-management and resourcefulness, many of their aims and interests can still be realised.

One of the main needs people with MS have if they are to follow the Wellness model and be self-managing as much as possible, is knowledge. This includes not only an understanding of MS and symptom management as it relates to them but also:

- developing appropriate coping strategies;
- an awareness of how they can keep themselves as healthy as possible;
- potential triggers that may cause a worsening of symptoms;
- their rights regarding benefits and employment;
- the different sources of help and support available to them;
- an understanding of when and who they should ask for help.

These broad themes are explored below so that nurses can advise their patients appropriately.

The law and disability

The Disability Discrimination Act 1995 prohibits discrimination against any individual with significant, long-term disability on the grounds of recruitment, promotion, transfer, training and development or the dismissal process. This act only applies to companies that employ 15 or more people. The act also makes it clear that service providers – for example shops, theatres, hospitals etc. – cannot refuse to serve an individual, nor offer a lower standard of service nor less favourable terms to someone with a disability, than they would to someone who is not disabled. From 2004 service providers must make reasonable alterations to their premises to enable equal access by people with a disability.

There are a few exceptions to this which centre largely on health and safety grounds. For example if the health and safety of the individual would be at risk or if by providing a service to someone with a particular disability other customers would be precluded from using the service (DFEE, 1995).

Employment

When someone is diagnosed with MS, one of the things they will have to consider is their current employment. People are understandably concerned about how their employers will react when told that they have MS, whether they will retain their ability to do their job and what their prospects for future employment are.

The answers to these queries will of course vary from person to person depending on their individual circumstances; however, there are some basic rights set out in the Disability Discrimination Act that can be used to clarify the situation somewhat.

An individual diagnosed with MS has no legal obligation to inform their employer although it is often more helpful for the individual if the employer is aware of potential problems. The vast majority of employers will do everything they can to support the person with MS. By informing the manager of their diagnosis, solutions to problems at work can be found. This also stops the manager jumping to (the wrong) conclusions about the problems the individual is experiencing. The employer is also then aware of their legal obligations towards the employee; any company with 15 or more employees is bound by the Disability Discrimination Act.

Whether an individual chooses to tell their colleagues at work is again a matter for them to decide depending upon their individual circumstances. People who have chosen not to tell their colleagues can find it makes work more difficult. Colleagues are often aware that the individual is having problems but without knowing the cause they may not fully appreciate the nature of the particular problems faced by that individual. The vast majority of people who have chosen to share their diagnosis with their work mates have been rewarded with support and understanding.

If someone with MS feels that they have been discriminated against because of their disability, they can access support through a number of different sources including the MS Society Helpline, Citizens' Advice Bureau, local job centre or trade union.

Often people with MS may require some adjustments to their workplace in order to allow them to continue to work. The Disability Discrimination Act ensures that employers must make 'reasonable adjustments' where necessary to allow the individual to stay in work. The local job centre will be able to put the individual in contact with the local disability employment advisor. They can then work with the individual and their employer towards providing an 'MS friendly' environment. Often equipment that may be needed (e.g. voice recognition software, specialist seating) can be loaned or the employer can apply for grants towards the cost of providing the equipment. Other relatively simple adjustments that can be made include flexible working hours, a car park space next to the entrance, easy access to the toilet etc. Most employers will do their best to accommodate the needs of people with MS.

The person with MS may feel that they want to change jobs or may find they reach a period of stability and wish to return to work. This can be difficult but again there are various options that the individual can explore.

The disability employment advisor at the job centre can be an invaluable resource. The individual must be realistic about their abilities and must be honest with any prospective employer. It is important that the individual answers any questions posed by their employer honestly as if information is withheld, the individual can be dismissed once the truth comes to light. However the individual is under no obligation to offer information that is not requested.

Voluntary work can provide a useful change of direction if income is not the driving force in trying to find some employment. Voluntary work provides the opportunity of meeting a challenge with short, flexible working hours in the company of others. It also allows the person with MS to give something to others rather than feeling that they are constantly on the receiving end.

Another option is for the individual to become self-employed. For example:

> MJ was working as an assistant in a busy chemist's shop. She was diagnosed with MS and subsequently left her job at the chemist. MJ then chose to retrain as a counsellor and is now self-employed with her own client base.

Retirement can be another option and can be a very positive move depending on the individual and their circumstances. Many people with MS find that fatigue is the most limiting factor as regards their employment. It often happens that while the individual is able to fulfil their responsibilities at work, they have no energy to do little more than sleep while at home. This is rarely satisfactory and puts an enormous strain on the person with MS and their family. Their quality of life and the extent of the role they can play within the family can become severely reduced. In these circumstances, many people choose to either reduce their hours or to take early retirement. Either of these options can allow the individual the freedom to pursue their interests outside work and to spend more quality time with their friends and family.

Benefits entitlement

Reduced financial income can be a very real problem for people with MS. At a time when their expenditure can increase (e.g. increased costs pertaining to transport, medications, diet and supplements etc.) people's income is often reduced. There are many different benefits that someone with MS may be eligible for. This is a complex and ever-changing area and the individual should be advised to contact their local Citizens' Advice Bureau or welfare rights office for assistance. People working in these offices are able to provide advice and support while the benefits claim is being submitted and processed. They can also ensure that the individual claims for all the relevant benefits depending on their particular circumstances. They are also usually able to visit people at home and help them fill in the claims forms.

A brief overview of some of the more commonly claimed benefits is included below.

Disability living allowance (DLA)

This is available to people who have been ill for at least 3 months and are expected to have problems for at least the next 6 months. It is not means tested, is tax-free and is only available to people less than 65 years old.

There are two components to DLA: Mobility and Care. Each of these is split into three different levels, i.e. low, middle and high. An award is made according to the individual's level of need.

Mobility allowance can be awarded on its own. If high-level mobility allowance is awarded for three years or more the individual can apply for a car (adapted if necessary); under the mobility scheme they are also exempted from having to pay car tax. Care allowance, at whatever level, is only awarded in conjunction with mobility allowance.

Disability working allowance (DWA)

This is paid to people in work to top up low wages for those who are at 'a disadvantage in getting a job'. The individual must have been on certain other benefits for at least eight weeks before getting a job. Not everyone is better off under this scheme and the individual should be advised to seek advice.

Incapacity benefit

From 2001 new claimants will be means tested against any private or occupational pension. If the individual receives more than £85 per week from their pension, their incapacity benefit will be reduced accordingly. Claimants must have been incapable of work for at least 6 months and have paid enough National Insurance contributions to be eligible for this benefit.

Driving

The individual with MS is not necessarily prevented from driving. They do, however, have an obligation to inform the driving and vehicle licensing authority (DVLA) that they have been diagnosed with MS. The individual will be asked to inform the DVLA if their condition deteriorates but will not be prevented from driving so long as they are safe to do so.

The individual should also tell their insurance company. If they have an accident and the insurance company find out that they have MS and have not informed them, then the individual will not be covered by their insurance policy. Insurance premiums should not be increased but the individual may have to 'shop around'. The MS Society can be very helpful in finding sympathetic insurers.

People with MS should also be advised to apply for a disabled parking badge from their local town hall. This allows them to park in spaces reserved for people with disabilities and this can prove invaluable in reducing fatigue etc. If the individual does not drive, they should be advised to contact their town hall anyway as many councils operate a scheme whereby the individual can apply for reduced taxi fares or a bus pass.

Lifestyle adaptations

Thus it can be seen that there are several different avenues that someone with MS can pursue to ensure that they fulfil their role at work as fully as they wish to. However in reality only a relatively small proportion of people with MS are actually in employment.

Having MS can allow people to focus on which things in life are really important to them. The next section of this chapter will examine various strategies that someone with MS can employ to ensure that they stay as well as possible and are able to make the most of their potential.

There is a lot that the individual can do to help themselves and it is the role of the nurse to teach patients some of the main points described in this chapter. The MS specialist nurse can also be invaluable in this role. Many MS nurses run courses for people newly diagnosed with MS to teach them about self-management (Brechin et al., 2001). The MS Society also run similar courses ('Getting to Grips'), often in conjunction with the MS specialist nurse, and local branches can provide more information about these.

Trigger factors

One of the main features of MS for many people is the recurring relapses and the uncertainty this can bring with it. While many relapses develop for no apparent reason, sometimes an exacerbation can be caused by certain trigger factors. These include:

- infection;
- prolonged exposure to heat;
- stress.

Infection

Many people with MS who develop an infection (bacterial or viral) often experience a worsening of their MS symptoms as a result (Rapp *et al.*, 1995; Panitch, 1997). While it is often difficult for individuals to avoid an infection, awareness of the potential problems can be helpful.

One of the most common infective triggers that can cause an exacerbation is a urinary tract infection. The nurse should ensure that the individual is aware of the symptoms of a urinary tract infection and that they subsequently take appropriate strategies to minimise their risk. For example, drinking two or more glasses of cranberry juice daily. See Chapter 6 for more detailed information about the management of bladder problems in MS. Often the first sign that someone with MS has a urinary tract infection is that their MS itself becomes a lot worse. Thus it is always worth screening someone with MS who is experiencing an exacerbation. A mid-stream specimen of urine will be sufficient to determine whether or not they have a urine infection.

It is not just a urinary tract infection that can cause a worsening of symptoms, any infection has this potential. If someone with MS develops an infection, they should be treated appropriately (i.e. given antibiotics as required). Steroids should not be given until the infection has settled down. As steroids act to suppress the body's natural immunity, any infection that is present will become much more vigorous. People often find that within a week or so of the infection settling down, any exacerbation of their MS has also settled.

Vaccinations are another way of minimising the risk of infection. This has been a grey area in the past and many people have been advised not to have vaccinations as it was thought that the vaccination itself may cause an exacerbation. The answer to this is still unclear although it is now thought that any vaccination is likely to cause far less problems than the infection itself would. Most clinicians would now recommend people with MS to have any necessary vaccinations (Panitch, 1997). This includes the 'flu-jab' each autumn.

Prolonged exposure to heat

The majority of people with MS find sustained high temperatures diffi-cult to cope with. Heat can leave the person with MS feeling weak, drained and fatigued. If the heat is prolonged, for example a hot spell during the summer, and appropriate precautions are not taken, the indi-vidual can experience a worsening of their MS.

Sensitivity to heat can cause problems in many different situations, for example a warm office can cause excess fatigue making it difficult for the individual to fulfil their workload; overheating during exercise can limit an individual's potential; an overheated hospital ward can make an indi-vidual's recovery more difficult etc.

However if the person with MS is made aware of the potential prob-lems that they may experience when they are somewhere hot, they will be able to develop some compensatory strategies (see Table 10.1).

It is worth noting at this point that not everyone with MS feels worse in the heat, a minority of people thrive in the heat and find cold temperatures particularly difficult to cope with. Common sense should prevail and the individual should take appropriate action to ensure they remain warm.

Table 10.1 Strategies to minimise heat related fatigue

- Avoid excessive heat, e.g. don't travel abroad at the peak season
- Don't have a hot bath prior to a period of planned activity
- Ensure hotel rooms/ office etc. have air conditioning or open windows
- Wear a wide-brimmed hat in the sun
- Carry and use a handheld fan
- If the temperature is particularly high, rub an ice cube on the pulse points at the wrist
- Drink plenty of iced drinks

Physical trauma and stress

There are many anecdotal reports of physical trauma (for example, a fall or car accident) causing a relapse. However a recent review of the research in this area concluded that there is no relationship between physical trauma and either the onset of MS or relapses (Goodin *et al.*, 1999). However the study concluded that it is quite likely that moderate levels of stress can cause exacerbations although more research is needed to confirm this relationship.

Certainly in practice, people with MS who experience a major stressor (e.g. bereavement, divorce etc.) often find that they subsequently experience a worsening of their MS symptoms. Equally prolonged and unmanaged stress can cause problems.

It is unrealistic to advise people with MS to avoid stress; unfortunately none of us is able to do this! However if the individual can learn to manage their stress more effectively then they should feel happier and more in control as well as reducing the risk of an exacerbation.

Techniques to manage stress and anxiety are many and varied and it is important that the individual chooses something that is appropriate for them. This could include simple breathing exercises, listening to a relaxation tape, practising T'ai Chi or yoga, reflexology or aromatherapy.

Diet and MS

People with MS often receive a lot of conflicting advice about diet. There has been a lot of credence given at various times in the past to specialised diets. In particular, this includes the gluten- or wheat-free diet, and low-fat or dairy-free diets. However it is now recognised that these more extreme diets are not particularly helpful. They can prove expensive, time-consuming and it is often difficult to obtain the correct balance of nutrients. There is also no scientific evidence that they are at all helpful.

This said some individuals do follow strict dietary regimes and state that they feel much better for doing so. Whether the benefits they feel are due to the diet or simply that their MS is currently stable or in remission is sometimes unclear; there is no scientific evidence to support gluten-free or dairy-free diets.

Advice for people with MS regarding diet is similar to that for anyone wishing to follow a healthy diet. The basic principles are listed below:

- High levels of fruit and fibre (at least 5 portions a day) which provide the vitamins A, C and E as well as potassium, magnesium, calcium and fibre.
- Reduce animal fats (i.e. saturated fats) although low-fat dairy products such as semi-skimmed milk, yoghurt, cottage cheese and eggs are fine.

They provide calcium, protein and vitamins D, E and B.

- Polyunsaturated fats should be deliberately included, e.g. sunflower oil and oily fish.
- Carbohydrates provide sustainable energy and should form a staple part of the diet; they are also an important source of fibre.
- Proteins, e.g. fish, chicken, beans etc., are necessary for muscle strength and as an energy source.

In essence this is a low-fat, high-fibre diet with plenty of fruit, vegetables and polyunsaturated fatty acids. Polyunsaturated fatty acids (PUFAs) are particularly important. They consist of linoleic acid and gamma linoleic acid and can only be obtained from the diet. PUFAs are one of the few food groups that research has shown to be helpful in ameliorating the effects of MS. Trials using 3–4 tablespoons of sunflower oil daily have demonstrated a significant reduction in relapse rate and severity as well as a slight slowing down of progression in people with mild relapsing-remitting MS (Dworkin *et al.*, 1984).

Many people with MS take supplements to a greater or lesser degree. If someone is following a healthy, balanced diet as described above, they shouldn't need to take any supplements. If someone with MS does feel strongly that they want to try something, the most useful are a multivitamin and either sunflower oil or evening primrose oil. However any supplements should be taken with care and the individual should be encouraged to discuss them with their doctor or a dietician prior to starting.

Dieticians can be very useful if people have particular problems and the nurse should ensure that anyone who needs the advice and support of a dietician is referred to the service.

Exercise

People with MS should be encouraged to pursue some form of exercise appropriate to their abilities. It has been shown that regular exercise over a period of time results in improved fitness despite the MS. The same study also showed that exercise can have a positive impact on factors related to quality of life (Petejan *et al.*, 1996). There are many different forms of exercise that can be pursued, for example yoga and swimming. Some people prefer to spend time in a gym (with appropriate instruction) or to walk a set distance each day. The type of exercise is not crucial, the important thing is that it is maintained over time, that the individual is able to achieve the chosen activity and that they enjoy the exercise. Physiotherapists are invaluable in advising people with regard to individual exercise programmes and the sort of exercises that would most meet their needs. Advice should always be sought as too much or the wrong sort of exercise can cause more problems than it solves.

Someone with MS who is keen to pursue an exercise programme should be encouraged in this, and should be reassured that while the process may be slow, it is possible for them to increase their stamina and fitness which in turn can make them feel better generally.

Coping with MS

People with MS face many challenges that must be coped with throughout their lives. The coping strategies that individuals develop will make an enormous difference to them and their families. Clinical experience suggests that people bring their existing coping strategies and attitudes to illness and disability with them. However, some people are able to improve their coping skills and maintain more effective strategies over time.

There are thought to be three different types of skills necessary to achieve effective, problem-focused coping:

- seeking information and support;
- taking appropriate action;
- identifying alternative rewards (Moos and Shaefer, 1984).

Problem-focused coping is a way of developing methods of coping that are directed towards changing the environment rather than changing oneself (which is called emotion-focused coping). The type of coping used by an individual depends on their personality, the level of support they have from their family and friends, and the amount of time they spend with friends and colleagues etc. (Murray, 1995).

Resources most commonly employed include self-reliance, optimism, humour, learning something new, thinking positively, wishing the problem would go away, and trying to keep life as normal as possible (A. Jalowic, cited in Murray, 1995).

Quality of life studies show that the factors which are most likely to cause a reduced quality of life include loneliness, fatigue, chronic pain, stressful life events and cognitive deficits (Ritvo et al., 1992).

It is the role of the nurse to talk to our patients and their families about MS and the way they cope with its impact. Individuals should be encouraged to review their coping strategies and determine whether or not these are the most effective for them. They may need the support of a psychologist, counsellor or MS nurse to do this. However effective symptom management and other simple strategies can also be effective – for example, helping the individual get out and about more. Input from the physiotherapist and occupational therapist can overcome most physical barriers. The nurse or occupational therapist may be able to advise the patient of local resources. These may include evening classes, voluntary work, social clubs, MS Society branch meetings, day centres etc. It is more often a problem of motivation and lack of confidence that restricts an individual's social activities than physical disability. However with support from family and friends and appropriate advice from the IDT, most people are able to socialise more. See, for example, Case study 7.

Case study 7

TT is a 45-year-old single man. He lives in a rural village and has enjoyed many countryside pursuits, particularly walking and birdwatching. He has had MS since he was 30 years old and has managed reasonably well until the last 3 years. He is now able to walk only a few yards with elbow crutches and has developed urinary incontinence over the last few months. As a result he has become more withdrawn and isolated. He no longer joins his friends on birdwatching expeditions and feels miserable whenever they try to include him in their discussions.

TT contacted his GP because of his incontinence and was assessed by the district nurses. They were able to teach him intermittent catheterisation, which solved his incontinence. The district nurses in turn referred TT to the community physiotherapist who spent several weeks with him. They were able to improve his stamina a little and do some confidence building with him. TT's mood gradually became a little more positive and he confided to the physiotherapist that he wished he could go birdwatching. His upper body strength and co-ordination were good and the physiotherapist suggested he use something like a quad bike to get around the fields.

TT began to see that it would be possible to rejoin his friends. He acquired a quad bike and equipped with a mobile phone and a pair of binoculars, was able to resume his social activities. His mood improved markedly and he was able to look at other activities in his life that he had thought were no longer open to him.

Thus it can be seen that by the appropriate members of the interdisciplinary team working together, with the person with MS central to the plan of care, then much can be achieved. Each individual will have different needs and problems and as a consequence will have evolved different coping strategies. By reflecting on these and looking at resources available to assist the individual social isolation can be lessened giving the individual a greater sense of control and restoring some structure and normality to their lifestyle.

The nurse is ideally placed to discuss various coping strategies with the individual and help them reflect on their effectiveness. The nurse also has an important role to play in educating the person with MS and their families on the importance of effective coping strategies and of the resources available to them (see Table 10.2). They should also be advised that there will be times when the person with MS feels low in mood and that this is a normal response and must be worked through. By focusing the interdisciplinary team on the problems relevant to the patient (e.g. fatigue, cognitive impairment, social isolation) and educating the patient and their family about the emotional impact of MS, the importance of maintaining social activities, and the many resources open to them, better coping strategies should follow.

Counter-productive coping strategies

Sometimes people with MS respond to a particular situation in a way that is counter-productive. If this is not recognised and resolved quickly, the pattern can be set and the individual may need help to resolve this pattern of behaviour.

Table 10.2 Example of the resources available to help people cope with MS

- Humour
- Optimism
- Positive thinking
- Support from family and friends
- Understanding of disease process
- Understanding of emotional impact on self and family
- Interdisciplinary team (particularly psychologist and MS specialist nurse)
- MS Society
- Resourcefulness
- Local activities/charities
- Voluntary sector
- Understanding that sometimes they will feel miserable

One of the most typical examples of inappropriate responses to a situation is described in the anxiety cycle (Wells, 1997). Many people, not just those with MS, become anxious in certain situations. People with MS often feel anxious in response to particular symptoms or thoughts related to their MS. For example they may experience the same symptom, which they developed last time they had a relapse, and become anxious that they are about to have another relapse. Thoughts that can trigger anxiety can be many and varied but tend to be of the 'What if ...?' variety. For example:

- 'What if my MS is relapsing or getting worse again?'
- 'What if people think I'm drunk when I go out?'
- 'What if I slur my words and can't give my presentation at work?'
- 'What if I feel dizzy again when I am crossing the road?'

Usually people are able to rationalise these fears and think problems through to their logical conclusion. For example, just because they are experiencing the same symptom again does not mean that a relapse is imminent. If a relapse does develop, they know that appropriate help and support will be available.

However, some people are unable to rationalise their fears and become drawn into a cycle of ever increasing anxiety.

Anxiety causes a physiological response within the body producing symptoms, which can include tiredness, blurred vision, a feeling of choking, needing the toilet, weakness in the legs, pins and needles etc. Many of these symptoms are similar to those of MS. This in turn confirms the individual's fears and the individual misinterprets the symptoms of anxiety for those of MS which in turn causes them to feel even more anxious, thus they can become stuck in an anxiety cycle (see Figure 10.1).

As mentioned above, anxiety can have a negative impact on an individual's MS and so the individual can find themselves in a situation where their symptoms of MS are exacerbated by anxiety.

It is important that people are taught how to mange their stress and anxiety better. It is also helpful if they understand what to expect in terms of symptoms and that by helping them express their fears and concerns, much progress can be made. The MS nurse or psychologist can facilitate the development of appropriate self-help strategies for people in this situation. Examples of useful self-help strategies are included in Table 10.3.

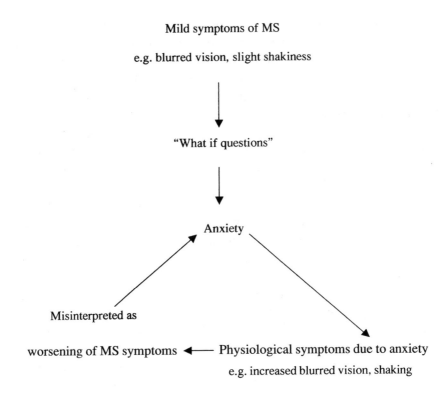

Mild symptoms of MS

e.g. blurred vision, slight shakiness

"What if questions"

Anxiety

Misinterpreted as

worsening of MS symptoms ◄——— Physiological symptoms due to anxiety

e.g. increased blurred vision, shaking

Figure 10.1 The anxiety cycle.

Table 10.3 Self-help strategies to combat anxiety

- Relaxation techniques
- Talk about fears and concerns
- Write down fears and concerns
- Challenge unrealistic fears and concerns
- Distraction, i.e. do something else enjoyable when feeling anxious
- Humour
- Remember other situations when you have succeeded
- Stop, pause and take a fresh look

Complementary therapies

Many people with MS will try some form of complementary therapy at some stage during their life with MS. This is often a response to a feeling that conventional medicine no longer has all the answers for them. Complementary therapies are based on a holistic model of care and often help the individual to feel more positive about themselves and their health. Using a complementary therapy is often a positive coping strategy and can help restore some sense of control to the individual.

These benefits aside, there are unfortunately few randomised control trials (i.e. the most robust form of scientific enquiry) that have been applied to complementary therapies and MS. In many instances there is little research of any type. While this means that there is little if any, scientific evidence that complementary therapies work, it also means that there is little evidence to prove that they don't work. Health professionals should therefore be advised to keep an open mind when discussing complementary therapies with patients. Indeed many health professionals including nurses, GPs and physiotherapists are themselves seeking to train in a particular therapy and to apply this to their sphere of practice. Almost 40% of GP practices in England now provide access to some form of complementary therapy for NHS patients (Owen *et al.*, 2001).

People with MS should be advised, however, on the importance of finding a reputable therapist and of choosing a therapy that best meets their needs. As there is little regulation of complementary therapists, virtually anyone can set up in practice as a practitioner regardless of whether or not they are actually qualified. There are various organisations and professional bodies that ensure practitioners who register with them achieve a certain standard and anyone wishing to find a reputable practitioner should be advised to contact them in the first instance.

Choosing a complementary therapy that suits can be very difficult. There is a lot of conflicting advice available, which is compounded by the lack of scientific evidence. This can lead to individuals trying a number of different therapies.

Complementary therapies are usually thought of as being safe and natural although this is not always borne out in practice. For example, some patients can have an adverse reaction after acupuncture or homeopathy; certain aromatherapy oils must not be used if the individual is pregnant or has epilepsy etc. Other complications may arise if an unqualified practitioner administers treatment or if the individual chooses complementary therapies at the expense of conventional medicine. Treatments can also prove expensive. People should be advised that they should choose a therapy and therapist that they feel comfortable with (preferably having first discussed this with their GP, neurologist or MS nurse). Ideally they should also speak to other clients of the therapist and ensure that they do not have to pay more than they feel they can afford. Many of the organisations listed in Appendix I can be a useful source of advice and further information. A brief overview of some of the more commonly used therapies is given below.

Herbalism

Herbs have been used to treat a multiplicity of disorders for several thousand years. Many of the herbs that were used have since been refined and now form the basis of 'modern medicine'. For example quinine which is used to treat malaria was originally derived from Cinchona bark and one of the best known is perhaps morphine which is derived from the opium poppy (Frost, 1992). Thus it can be seen that some of the herbs prescribed by a herbalist potentially have as many side effects (and benefits) as conventional medications. It is also quite possible for any herbs that are recommended to interact with prescription medications. There have been no studies examining the effect of herbalism in the context of MS and people should be advised to proceed with caution and ask the advice of their GP or neurologist in the first instance.

Homeopathy

This is the use of extremely diluted substances that are usually administered as tablets or drops. Homeopaths, as do all complementary therapists, take a full history from the individual, which takes account of all aspects of their life so that they are then able to match the remedy to the individual's needs.

Acupuncture

Acupuncture has obscure origins dating back over thousands of years. It is the Chinese that have developed the philosophy and principles of acupuncture, which is based on a philosophy of interconnectedness and balance. Each individual has three different types of energy, i.e. jing, shen and qi (pronounced 'chi'). Qi represents the individual's life force and is adversely affected by ill health, causing a disturbance in the balance of energies.

Acupuncture involves the insertion of very fine needles into specific points on the body which are chosen depending on the particular problems the individual is experiencing. It is believed that this acts to restore the balance of energies (Trevelyan, 1993).

Again there are no studies examining the benefits (or otherwise) of acupuncture in MS. However its use is becoming more widespread within the NHS and it may well have an increasing part to play in the management of specific symptoms such as pain.

Massage

Massage is a systematic form of touch that uses certain manipulations of the soft tissues to promote comfort and healing (Carruthers, 1992). Massage is also very relaxing and can be a very effective stress reliever. A randomised control trial comparing two groups of people with MS, one of whom received twice weekly massages while the other received none, showed significant results in terms of reduced anxiety and improved mood with increased self-esteem and body image (Hernandez-Reif *et al.*, 1998).

Aromatherapy

Aromatherapy may be combined with massage or used in isolation. It is the use of essential plant oils to create a mood or to ease a particular body system. The oils are very concentrated and should not be applied directly to the skin. If the oils are to be massaged in they should be diluted in a carrier or base oil such as grape seed oil or almond oil.

Essential oils can also be added to bathwater, to a tissue or vaporised using a room burner. Different oils are chosen depending on the needs of the individual, for example lavender and camomile are relaxing while orange and peppermint are uplifting. Care should be taken, however, as some oils are contraindicated in certain circumstances, e.g. if the individual is pregnant or has epilepsy. A reputable practitioner should always be chosen.

Reflexology

This is a form of therapy that is based on the principle that energy zones connect all the different parts of the body. Stimulation of specific areas on the feet is thought to release energy by unblocking energy channels, which have been adversely affected by the individual's ill health.

Many people find reflexology very relaxing and from anecdotal evidence it seems to be one of the more helpful forms of complementary therapies for people with MS. There has been some research done which demonstrated significant improvements in altered sensation, bladder dysfunction, muscle strength and spasticity compared to the control group (Siev-Ner *et al.*, 1997).

Relaxation

As mentioned earlier, stress and anxiety can cause an exacerbation of MS and reduce the individual's ability to cope if left unmanaged. While avoidance of stress is impossible, strategies to manage stress should be actively sought. There are many different forms that relaxation can take, e.g. breathing exercises, visualisation, focused muscle relaxation, meditation etc. The individual must find a method that they feel comfortable with. Two of the simpler methods of relaxation are outlined in Box 10.1.

Many people also find listening to relaxation tapes can be very helpful. The MS Society has a good selection of tapes as do many health food shops and book shops.

T'ai Chi and yoga

While not exactly complementary therapies, T'ai Chi and yoga can be very helpful for people with MS. They both require the individual to make slow, measured movements and are able to promote balance and strength. Both also have an element of relaxation built in which is equally beneficial.

A study of people with MS participating in an eight week T'ai Chi course (two x 1 hour lessons a week) found that the participants improved with regard to walking speed and flexibility as well as vitality, social functioning and mental health (Husted *et al.*, 1999). Certainly on an anecdotal level, a number of people with MS have taken up T'ai Chi or yoga and found it very helpful in improving their balance and muscle control.

Hyberbaric oxygen

This is quite a popular treatment used by a number of people with MS. It involves sitting in a pressure chamber while the pressure is increased gradually and subsequently decreased. Each session lasts approximately two hours and the individual also has to use an oxygen mask during the session. The tanks are the same as those used by deep-sea divers who have depressurised too quickly and developed 'the bends'. There are hyperbaric tanks at MS therapy centres around the country (see Appendix I). It is thought that by forcing oxygen at high pressures into body tissues some benefits will be felt. A review (Kleijnen and Knipschield, 1995) of controlled studies into the use of hyberbaric oxygen therapy found no scientific evidence that it is beneficial. However, anecdotally many people do report feeling better and in particular have noted an

Box 10.1 Two simple relaxation exercises

Breathing exercise
- Find a quiet place to sit or lie in and ensure you are comfortable and will be undisturbed.
- Take a deep, slow breath in, hold it for a moment and breathe slowly out again.
- Check that you are breathing from your diaphragm by feeling the rise and fall of your abdomen with your hands.
- Let your breathing come naturally, you may wish to close your eyes to aid concentration.

As you breathe in and out imagine that your body is beginning to slow down; let your breathing slow down and concentrate on a feeling of calm.

Focused muscle relaxation
Find somewhere comfortable and quiet to sit; ensure you are away from distractions and will not be disturbed. Sit with your hands resting on your lap, uncross your legs and loosen any tight clothing.

Begin with the breathing exercises and allow your body to slow down a little before beginning.

- Push your heels into the ground, feel the tension in the calves and thighs ... hold ... and let go. Repeat.
- Clench your buttocks together ... hold ... let go. Repeat.
- Push the small of your back into the chair ... feel your abdomen tighten ... hold ... let go. Repeat.
- Clench your hands into a fist ... hold ... let go. Repeat.
- Lift your shoulders slightly ... hold ... then drop. Lift them up higher ... hold ... drop. Lift them up to your ears ... hold ... drop.
- Clench the teeth together ... hold ... let them go. Clench them again ... now let go so that the jaw drops and the mouth opens slightly. Feel your tongue resting gently in your mouth.
- Pull your mouth into a wide smile ... hold ... let go. Repeat.
- Screw up your eyes tightly ... hold ... let go. Repeat.
- Frown and wrinkle up the skin between your eyebrows ... hold ... let go. Repeat.

When you have finished sit quietly and calmly for a few minutes enjoying the sensation of relaxation.

With thanks to Lorraine Lawton, Sapphire Nurse for allowing the reproduction of part of her patient information leaflet 'Relax and enjoy life'.

improvement in bladder and bowel symptoms. Many also found the peer support gained by attending the centres invaluable.

The treatment needs to be carried out over a prolonged period of time and can be quite costly. As with all complementary therapies, individuals should be advised to discuss it with their doctor or MS nurse initially.

This gives a very brief overview of some of the most commonly tried complementary therapies. What is needed is scientifically sound research that demonstrates the effectiveness (or otherwise) of these therapies (Huntley and Ernst, 2000). However, for the present many people with MS gain a great deal of benefit in terms of emotional well being and should not be dissuaded from trying a particular therapy provided they proceed with caution.

CHAPTER 11

Complications and management of severe MS

Introduction

While many people with MS are able to fulfil the majority of their responsibilities, roles and personal cares, a significant proportion of people will become severely disabled. When this happens, the MS takes over their lives and that of their family, it affects every action they take, be it going to visit a friend or eating a meal.

The care of someone with severe MS poses health professionals with a huge challenge. The affected individual can be physically and emotionally draining to care for. It is also this group of people that are seen most often by health professionals, certainly within the hospital setting and often in the community as well.

The objectives of caring for someone who is severely disabled by MS are to provide effective symptom management, promote comfort, provide emotional support, prevent complications and improve the quality of life for the individual and their family as far as possible. These aims fall within the scope of palliative care. Many people with MS and even some health professionals associate palliative care only with terminal cancer. However the principles can be applied equally to encompass the needs of someone with severe disability. Indeed many hospices are now providing services for people with severe MS and other chronic disabling conditions. This chapter will endeavour to discuss the symptoms and possible complications that are usually only seen in someone with severe MS and will go on to explore the wider needs of the individual and their family.

Spasticity

Many people with MS will develop some degree of spasticity. However individuals with severe MS are more likely to have a degree of spasticity that adversely affects their quality of life. They are also prone to developing contractures, which can be a complication of under-managed, severe spasticity.

The term spasticity is derived from the Greek *spastikos* which means to tug or draw. The definition that is most often quoted is that devised by Lance in 1980:

> Spasticity is a motor disorder characterised by a velocity-dependent increase in tonic stretch reflexes ('muscle tone') with exaggerated tendon jerks, resulting from hyper excitability of the stretch reflex, as one component of the upper motor neurone syndrome.

Simplifying this definition, spasticity occurs as a result of increased muscle tone, which in turn causes stiffness. It is an upper motor neurone syndrome and can be demonstrated during a neurological examination by brisk reflexes (i.e. hyperexcitable reflexes). In practical terms the individual's limbs feel very stiff and exhibit varying degrees of resistance to movement. Many people describe the affected limb(s) as feeling heavy, and if they are still mobile, as though they are wading through deep water when walking.

The pathophysiology of spasticity is very complex. As mentioned previously, it is a feature of an upper motor neurone disorder. The upper motor neurones are the nerve tracts that descend down from a specific area in the brain through to the spinal cord where they link, via synapses, with the interneuronal networks within the spine. The most commonly affected upper motor neurones in spasticity are the parapyramidal tracts. Most of these arise in the brainstem and link with the interneuronal network in the spinal cord that controls the stretch reflex and the flexor and extensor reflexes (Sheean, 1998a). In MS, the plaques that occur as a result of demyelination form somewhere along the length of the descending tract (i.e. within the brain or more commonly the spinal cord) and thus disrupt the pathway between the central nervous system and the muscles. Therefore 'messages' being transmitted from the spinal cord to the muscles become scrambled, slowed or completely blocked. The muscles respond by becoming overactive or excitable, which in turn leads to an increase in tone and stiffness.

People with moderate–severe MS also often experience spasms. These are painful and involuntary muscle contractions within the affected limb. They are often elicited when the individual tries to move or is moved by their carer(s), although a number of other factors can aggravate both spasms and spasticity (see Table 11.1).

Table 11.1 Aggravating factors in spasticity

- Movement and handling
- Infection
- Inappropriate seating
- Poor posture
- Warmth
- Pain
- Constipation
- Stress
- Pressure sores
- Tight, ill-fitting clothes or orthoses

Impact of spasticity on the individual

Severe spasticity can have a profound effect on the individual's quality of life and on their ability to fulfil the simple daily tasks that they would wish to (Melia, 1998). Spasticity can be painful and uncomfortable; it can make transferring someone or handling them in any way very fraught. Thus it can be seen that spasticity can impact on every aspect of an individual's life; including their level of mobility, their dexterity, bladder management, sexuality, hygiene needs, sleep, comfort and posture etc. (Thompson, 1998).

One of the complications of severe spasticity can be contractions which occur when there is a fixed shortening of the muscle leading to a reduced range of movement in that limb. Contractions are not solely the result of spasticity or spasms but may also be caused by continual poor positioning of a muscle in a shortened position (i.e. flexed). The physiotherapist is central to preventing the development of contractions by providing advice with respect to correct positioning and exercise (passive or otherwise).

Contractions in particular can cause many problems. As the affected individual is no longer able to straighten their limb(s), they may experience difficulty sitting in a wheelchair, maintaining a comfortable position, sleeping etc. As contractions affect the individual's posture and position they can also result in an increased risk of pressure sores.

Some individuals develop adductor spasms of the upper thighs. This results in the upper legs becoming very stiff and very difficult to separate. This in turn leads to problems maintaining the individual's hygiene needs, elimination can also pose particular problems, regardless of whether or not the individual is catheterised.

Carers, be they a family member or a professional, will also be greatly affected by the problems caused by spasticity. The spasms and stiffness can make handling and transferring the individual very difficult and potentially painful, which in turn distresses the carer. Difficulty using a wheelchair may mean that the individual becomes effectively house-bound and again this has a profound impact on all concerned.

Management and treatment of spasticity can only be effected through an interdisciplinary approach.

Management of spasticity and prevention of complications

When treating spasticity it is important to appreciate in the first instance what the aims of treatment are – i.e. is the treatment intended to improve the individual's function; to reduce their pain; to prevent complications; or to allow their carers to meet the individual's needs more fully. In mild–moderate spasticity treatment may be inappropriate as many people with MS use the increased tone in their legs to compensate for the underlying weakness so allowing them to walk. If the increased tone is resolved, the individual may find that as a result they are much weaker and consequently find it difficult to walk. However, in severe MS this is unlikely to be the case, most people will be wheelchair bound or able to walk just a very short distance with assistance. In most cases the aims of treatment will include all those mentioned above. The spasticity and/or spasms can rarely be fully resolved but if the individual can gain some relief from the pain and discomfort and find they can move and transfer more easily, maintain their elimination and hygiene needs and, hopefully, prevent contractions from forming, then the treatment can be said to be successful, at least in part.

Resolution of aggravating factors

Before starting any treatment regime it is important that the individual is assessed with respect to the presence or otherwise of any factors that may be aggravating the spasticity. For example if there is a focus of infection this should be treated; any faecal impaction should likewise be resolved. Any pain or irritation should be managed appropriately.

It is also vital that a full assessment by the physiotherapist and occu-pational therapist is carried out at this stage. They will be able to advise the individual and their carer with respect to correct positioning and handling. They can review the individual's wheelchair and seating position and make adjustments as required or refer the individual to a wheelchair clinic for assessment.

The physiotherapist and occupational therapist can also advise the individual and their family about fatigue management, aids and appliances for the home, and an appropriate exercise routine.

By treating any aggravating factors in this way the worst effects of the spasticity can be resolved before any more complicated treatment is instigated.

Medication

There are various oral medications that can be used to ease spasticity. Medication should always be the first-line choice and is discussed in more detail in Chapter 5, however, in severe spasticity, medication alone is often ineffective or insufficient and other modes of treatment must be considered.

Cannabis

It is known from anecdotal evidence and a few small-scale studies that cannabis can be effective in reducing spasticity and spasms. (It is also likely that it helps to ease other symptoms of MS including tremor, pain, and some bladder problems (Iverson, 2000).) A significant number of people with MS use cannabis to provide relief from these symptoms although this practice remains illegal at the present time. At the time of writing, a large scale, multi-centred trial using cannabis oil, a cannabis derivative, and placebo has begun. It is hoped to include approximately 660 participants in over 40 centres initially. The study is hoping to demonstrate a significant reduction in spasticity with secondary outcomes including control of pain and urinary dysfunction (Dyer, 2001). It is hoped eventually, that if the trial is successful in demonstrating the positive effects of cannabis, it will be licensed for use by people with MS and will be available on prescription.

Other types of treatment

In moderate–severe MS it is often difficult to manage spasticity by oral anti-spasticity agents alone. In addition side effects of oral medication may make their use at the required dose untenable. Other options are outlined below.

Botulinum toxin

Most spasticity is relatively localised and effective reduction of spasticity can be achieved by directing treatment just at the affected muscle group. Botulinum is produced by the bacterium *Clostridium botulinum* and is one of the most potent neurotoxins known. Botulinum toxin causes paralysis and, used selectively, injected into individual muscles, it is known to have a therapeutic effect on a number of other conditions as well as spasticity in MS (e.g. facial dystonia, some movement disorders, and childhood cerebral palsy).

There are seven different types of botulinum toxin and the type currently in routine clinical use is known as type A (Davis and Barnes, 2000). Botulinum toxin works by preventing the release of acetylcholine at the junction between the nerve and the muscle. Acetylcholine is the means by which the nerve transmits its message to the muscle effecting contraction (or relaxation) of the muscle. Thus by preventing the muscle from receiving any instruction from the nervous system, the muscle is effectively paralysed and any increased tone resulting from over-stimulation, as in MS, is lost. Its use to reduce spasticity significantly was first demonstrated in 1990 (Snow *et al.*, 1990).

Botulinum toxin is given by injection, the toxin being diluted in normal saline, and injected directly into the affected muscle(s). The toxin spreads within the muscle and the effect is usually seen within 2–3 days of the injection and lasts 3–6 months. Due to the fact that the effect of botulinum toxin is temporary, repeat injections are required to maintain the benefits.

Despite botulinum being a potent neurotoxin, side effects are very rare and it is generally well tolerated. A very few people can develop flu-like symptoms but the vast majority of people experience no ill effects. In the long term approximately 5% of people receiving the injection will cease to gain benefit from them as they develop antibodies to the type A toxin. Work is going on to develop type B toxin to the stage where it is licensed for use in this context (Barnes, 1999). It is known that type B toxin is equally as effective as type A and can provide an alternative in people who do not respond to type A (Cullis *et al.*, 1998).

In practical terms, botulinum toxin injections can be a simple and effective way to reduce the problems caused by severe spasticity and to improve comfort for the individual and potentially reduce the need for oral anti-spasticity agents. Thus the risk of developing contractures and all the associated problems is also much reduced. Its primary use in MS must be with people who have already lost function in the affected limb, as due to the mode of action of the toxin, muscle function is not restored. Despite this, individuals can find the injections make a big improvement to their quality of life.

Case study 8

MG is a retired designer. She has had MS for 25 years. After a period of some ten years, when she was lost to follow up, she presented at a general neurology clinic with flexion contractures in both her legs. These were causing her a great deal of pain and discomfort. The carers were finding it very difficult to keep her clean and comfortable and to maintain her urethral catheter. MG was also finding it very difficult to maintain a comfortable sitting position for any length of time and so was spending most of her time in bed.

After careful assessment by the neurologist, physiotherapist and occupational therapist, MG was given botulinum toxin injections in the appropriate muscles in both legs. Within a few days and with input from the physiotherapists and occupational therapists, MG was able to sit in her wheelchair for three hours at a time, she was much more comfortable, with little pain and the carers found it much easier to meet her hygiene needs. MG has the injections repeated six monthly and the initial improvements have been maintained.

The importance of physiotherapy in association with botulinum toxin injections cannot be overstressed. The physiotherapist will use a combination of stretching exercises and possibly splinting to maintain muscle length (Sheean, 1998b). The physiotherapist can also advise the individual and their carers about the best way to position and transfer them as this can change once the spasticity has been reduced. The physiotherapist may also show the carers how to use passive exercises to maintain muscle length and range of movement after discharge. The use of toxin without physiotherapy is likely to prove much less effective than a combined approach although a randomised controlled trial to study this has yet to be carried out.

Phenol block

This was used quite commonly in the past but has largely been superseded today, although it can still be an effective way to reduce spasticity in the legs of people with severe disability. Phenol is injected intrathecally, thus blocking any nerve transmissions below the injected site. Phenol often damages the sacral nerves and therefore may potentially result in urinary and faecal incontinence, and loss of sensation (Werring and Thompson, 1998). This in turn increases the individual's risk of developing pressure sores.

However if used selectively in individuals for whom other options have proven ineffective and who have already developed severe disability, loss of bladder and bowel control, no useful motor function in their legs and are not, nor are likely to be, sexually active, it can provide some relief from the problems of severe spasticity.

Intrathecal baclofen

Intrathecal baclofen or the baclofen pump is gaining in popularity. However the fact that it involves surgical implantation of a pump mechanism with a catheter connecting the pump to the intrathecal space, the somewhat prohibitive cost and the ongoing support and maintenance required, means that their widespread use has been less than it might have been. This said, a baclofen pump can provide some individuals with significant relief from spasticity.

When baclofen is given orally, large doses are often needed to achieve an effect. Side effects are common and can include drowsiness, weakness and potential liver damage. By administering baclofen directly into the cerebrospinal fluid within the spinal cord, benefits can be obtained using much smaller doses. Trial and insertion of baclofen pumps only takes place within specialised units. The majority of nurses working with people with MS will not be directly involved in the care or management of patients undergoing this procedure. However patients under your care may be referred for a baclofen pump or may wish to know more about this as one of the options available to them. To this end, an overview of the procedure and management of the pump follows.

The type of person who would most benefit from intrathecal baclofen is someone with MS who has severe lower limb spasticity, which impacts significantly on their quality of life. Other more conservative treatments must have been tried without success. The use of a baclofen pump also requires the individual and their partner or carer to have an appreciable understanding of its maintenance and potential problems and solutions (Weeks, 1997 cited in Kamansek, 1999).

Once an individual has been assessed by their neurologist and has chosen to use intrathecal baclofen, referral to a specialist centre will be necessary. The first step is a trial of intrathecal baclofen. A lumbar puncture is performed and a bolus dose of intrathecal baclofen administered. In this way the most effective dose can be established while the individual is carefully monitored for any adverse reactions.

Once the test dose has been completed and the patient and doctor are satisfied that a baclofen pump is the best treatment option available, the individual will be admitted to hospital for insertion of the pump. The pump (which is 3 inches in diameter) is sited subcutaneously in the abdominal area and care is taken to ensure that clothing, wheelchair arms etc. will not cause discomfort once the pump is in situ. During the surgery required for pump insertion, a catheter is placed in the appropriate position and the rest of the catheter is then tunnelled under the skin to the abdomen where it is attached to the pump.

The patient is closely monitored during the initial postoperative period as would be expected. The insertion site should be kept clean and dry and protected from any mishandling. While the patient is in hospital recovering from the surgery, the most effective dose of baclofen can be determined and the pump set to deliver this amount on discharge.

The pump consists of a refillable drug reservoir and the amount of baclofen pumped from the reservoir into the catheter and subsequently the intrathecal space is controlled by a microprocessor. The microprocessor is powered by a battery with a life of approximately 3–5 years depending on the rate of drug delivery (Kamansek, 1999). The pump can be programmed externally and stores information that the doctor can review by use of the external programmer. This also allows the doctor to alter the dose of baclofen that is being administered remotely.

All pumps are fitted with an alarm (usually a soft high-pitched beeping sound) that will sound if the pump needs refilling, if the battery is low or if the pump has stopped working. The drug reservoir within the pump is easily refilled by injection, this is usually necessary every 6–8 weeks. When the battery needs replacing this requires a further surgical procedure.

Insertion of a baclofen pump can make a huge difference to suitable individuals. The stiffness and spasms they have been experiencing can be greatly reduced. This means that they experience much less pain and are generally more comfortable. The individual is able to sleep better which makes them and their partner feel better generally. The person with MS is also much less likely to develop pressure sores and may become more independent as they meet more of their own self-care needs.

Potential side effects

Intrathecal baclofen is generally well tolerated. Its effects are reversible and non-destructive (as opposed to a phenol block, for example). There are of course the usual risks associated with undergoing any surgical procedure and an anaesthetic. Side effects specific to the pump implantation include infection, accumulation of fluid in the area in which the pump is sited, or CSF leakage and associated headaches. It is also possible for the catheter to leak or kink or become disconnected which may require corrective surgery, as would failure of the pump or one of its components.

There is also the potential for overdose, which can cause serious problems. However overdose in this context is very rare and has generally been related to procedural errors (Kamansek, 1999).

It is vital that anybody who it is thought may benefit from a baclofen pump has the procedure, potential benefits, potential side effects and subsequent follow up fully explained to them. They will need plenty of opportunity to ask questions and discuss their fears with a well-informed health professional.

Surgical treatment of spasticity

Surgery is very much a last resort and tends to be used only in the most intractable cases when all other options have failed and the individual has developed contractures that adversely affect their quality of life. The aim of surgery within the central nervous system is to reduce contractures by interrupting the stretch reflex in order to reduce the amount of impulses transmitted to the muscles, which are causing the over excitation. Alternatively increasing the inhibitory transmissions relating to the affected muscle can also be helpful (Smythe and Peacock, 2000). This tends to be performed only in specialist centres.

Peripheral surgery consists of the excitatory nerve, which is transmitting impulses to the affected muscle, being cut. Central surgery includes a number of techniques, one of the most common of which is dorsal rhizotomy. This involves 25–50% of the affected nerve roots being identified and cut within the spinal cord in the area between L2–S2. This may well result in weakness and is obviously permanent. Functional control cannot be restored but ease from the problems of spasticity may be achieved (Conference Report, 2000).

The tendons attaching the muscle to the bone are much more commonly the target for surgery. If someone has developed contractures, the tendons can become foreshortened and may need to be lengthened or even cut to allow the affected limb to be straightened and so allow a resolution of the contractures.

Early treatment of spasticity should prevent the need for such a drastic intervention as surgery.

In summary spasticity and its complications can cause pain, discomfort, lack of sleep, pressure sores, and adversely affect the quality of life of the person with MS and their family. There are several different treatments available but all require a combined approach by the doctor, physiotherapist, occupational therapist, and nurse. In this way the impact of spasticity can be significantly reduced and the potential complications averted.

Tremor

Tremor is a relatively common complaint in MS but tends to be at its worst in people with severe MS.

Tremor in MS is different from that seen in other neurological conditions for example Parkinson's disease, in that it is not a resting tremor. There are two types of tremor that may be experienced in MS. The tremor experienced by most people is typically triggered by any goal directed movement, e.g. reaching for a cup. This is known as 'intention tremor'. The other type of tremor that may be seen in people with MS is known as 'postural tremor'. This can affect the head, neck, trunk and limbs (head tremor is known as titubation). Any sort of tremor experienced by someone with MS has the potential to be severely disabling and is, unfortunately, often difficult to treat (Alusi *et al.*, 1999).

Postural tremor

This can involve almost the whole body and can severely limit an individual's ability to walk or care for themselves, for example:

> FT is a 62-year-old lady who has had MS for 32 years. She has a concentration of plaques in the cerebella region and suffers from severe postural tremor. F has a Zimmer frame but finds this very difficult to use as whenever she moves from a sitting position the tremor occurs with increasing amplitude so that her whole body shakes.

Intention tremor

This occurs when an individual tries to move towards something. It is often worse relative to the degree of precision required to complete the intended movement. This type of tremor can be hugely frustrating for the individual and at its worst can mean they are unable to achieve any useful movement with their arms. The movement of the arms can even be so violent as to cause the person injury, for example:

> JF is 36 years old and has had MS for 12 years. She has a severe intention tremor. J was trying to push her glasses up on one occasion but due to the violence of her tremor she missed her glasses and caused some bruising to the side of her face.

Treatment

Unfortunately tremor can be very difficult to treat satisfactorily. The most commonly used medications are beta-blockers, usually propanolol. Other medications that may be used include primidone, clonazepam, and hyoscine (Compston, 1998d). Some people also find that cannabis can be helpful in calming tremor (Clifford, 1983) although to date, there have been no large-scale trials to examine this claim. However medications are rarely satisfactory in terms of hoped for outcomes.

Patients usually adapt to some extent by using both arms, holding the affected arm against something while reaching with the other, or restraining their arms to prevent injury (Alusi *et al.*, 1999). The occupational therapist can be very helpful. They can advise the individual with respect to choreographing tasks and providing aids and adaptations to allow them to achieve tasks they could not manage otherwise. The occupational therapist may also use specially designed weights around the individual's wrist. The idea of this is that the force of the weight will counteract the force of the tremor so allowing the individual to regain some function in that arm. Unfortunately this too is of limited value, particularly if there is underlying weakness in the limb or if the tremor is severe.

Neurosurgery is very much a last resort, thalamotomy has been shown to relieve tremor in upwards of 65% of patients although tremor returns in about 20% of people within 12 months. Functional improvement with meaning to the patient is limited (Alusi *et al.*, 1999). Thalamotomy involves major surgery and the individual may well find they take some considerable time to recover after the operation. Other reported complications include worsening gait, hemiparesis, dysarthia, epilepsy, depression, and lethargy.

Any surgery of this type will only be carried out in specialist centres and patients will be carefully selected and counselled prior to any intervention.

People with MS who are trying to cope with severe tremor will need a lot of support and advice from the interdisciplinary team. The only workable solution may be to implement a package of care via social services so that paid carers can help the individual maintain their activities of daily living. Under these circumstances the patient and their family may need a great deal of support.

Dysphagia

Dysphagia, or difficulty swallowing, is common in MS. In mild–moderate MS this is usually first noticed when the individual starts coughing and spluttering when drinking. As with the majority of symptoms in MS, fatigue, heat and stress can all make it worse.

Input from the speech and language therapist is most important. They are able to make a full assessment of the problem and can advise on simple techniques to make swallowing easier. These may include:

- maintaining an upright posture with chin tucked in;
- alternating liquids with solids;
- using thickening agents in liquids;
- warming or cooling food to stimulate the swallowing reflex;
- taking small mouthfuls;
- eating little and often;
- moistening food with gravy etc.;
- liquidising food (Schapiro *et al.*, 1997).

People who have developed severe MS may also find their swallowing becomes very difficult. They may lose their gag reflex and ultimately may aspirate food or saliva. Speech therapists are able to assess the extent of any such problems either by a bedside examination or videofluoroscopy. A videofluoroscopy consists of observing the passage of a radio-opaque substance, drunk by the individual, from the mouth through the oesophagus. In this way the speech therapist can observe the exact nature of any problems and is also able to see if there is any aspiration occurring.

Aspiration of food, fluids, or saliva can be potentially fatal. This can be a particular risk in individuals who already have weakened respiratory muscles due to enforced inactivity as a result of the extent of their disability. This is aggravated by the fact that people can aspirate 'silently', i.e. because they have no gag reflex food, fluids and saliva can slip down the trachea without the individual or their carers being aware. This then acts as a focus of infection and the individual can very easily develop a severe chest infection.

Treatment

When routine measures such as those outlined above fail and the dysphagia is severe and ongoing, with a real risk of aspiration, percutaneous endoscopic gastrostomy (PEG) must be considered. Insertion of a PEG involves insertion of a tube through the abdomen into the stomach, which is guided into place by use of an endoscopy tube.

A PEG should also be considered in individuals who are steadily losing weight or are at risk of becoming malnourished, as they are too fatigued to eat enough calories during any 24-hour period.

Case study 9

CJ was a 45-year-old lady who was diagnosed with MS when she was 17 years old. CJ was severely disabled and unable to meet any of her own care needs. Despite support and advice from the speech and language therapist and dieticians, C's sister was unable to give her enough food to maintain her weight above 52kg. (Her target weight as recommended by the dietician was 55kg.) C was able to chew and swallow her food only very slowly, and quickly became tired. She had also had several quite frightening choking episodes over the previous six months. When C attended the appointment with her neurologist, her sister voiced her concerns about C's weight. The neurologist also had reports from the dietician and speech therapist. After further discussion with C and her sister, C was admitted for assessment.

During her admission C's problems were fully assessed and the idea of a PEG was discussed with her and her sister. Although initially not very keen on the idea, C realised that she could not continue indefinitely as she had been doing and agreed to the procedure.

C had an uneventful insertion of her PEG and was discharged home a week later. The speech therapist had agreed that C could continue with some soft oral diet and the dietician had organised a feeding regime via the PEG to be given overnight while C slept.

Within two months C was maintaining her target weight. She was also feeling better generally and her communication had improved a little. She was enjoying her oral diet and felt relieved that there was no longer any pressure on her to 'eat up'. Consequently she felt much less tired and more in control.

Support required

Broaching the subject of PEG insertion with someone with severe swallowing problems and their carers can produce a range of emotions and concerns. Initially, many people find it difficult to accept that they need one. For many the idea that they cannot eat anything any more is devastating. Often food is one of the few sociable activities they can still join in with. Ideally the necessity for a PEG should be broached before it becomes a matter of urgency. If the individual can have it inserted while they can still manage some oral diet, it is much more acceptable and can be seen as a positive move. Whatever the circumstances, the individual and their family will need a great deal of support, reassurance and information. This, of course, is part of the nursing care required. The support and advice needs to be ongoing after discharge and district nurses will be closely involved at this stage.

PEGs are usually well tolerated but complications can arise, for example the PEG may come out of place. Alternatively, the feeding regime may be too rich initially and cause profuse diarrhoea (particularly if the individual hasn't been eating much in the weeks/months leading up to PEG insertion); however, as a general rule, the benefits outweigh the disadvantages.

Optimal nutritional intake can:

- promote skin integrity;
- aid healing of any pressure sores;
- possibly result in some general improvement;
- allow correct and easy administration of medication via the tube;
- reduce fatigue;
- ensure a much reduced risk of aspiration;
- allow more time for social activities/therapy during the day;
- be hidden under clothing during the day (after Annoni *et al.*, 1998).

Skin care

People who are seriously disabled as a result of MS are at risk of developing pressure sores. Risk factors include the following.

Contractures

These make positioning difficult and may cause shearing when moving the individual. They can also cause increased pressure in one area for example, hip or heel, due to spasms and difficulty in finding alternative positions that the individual can be comfortable with.

Poor nutrition and hydration

If the individual is having problems swallowing, they may not be taking in enough calories or fluids to maintain optimal skin health and healing.

Reduced sensation

People with MS often have areas of reduced sensation or even numbness. These areas can be quite extensive in advanced MS, which in practical terms means that the individual is unable to feel pain or discomfort – the usual warning signs that would make people change position.

Immobility

Even if the individual is able to feel and express pain, they may be unable to change position themselves and have to wait until their carer is able to assist them.

Inappropriate seating/mattress

It is important that the individual is assessed by the occupational therapists and/or district nurses for their wheelchair seating and need for a pressure-relieving mattress. If the individual uses other seating during the day, this should also be assessed and the individual and their carers advised appropriately.

Elimination dysfunction

If the individual is incontinent of urine and/or faeces and the skin is often damp then the risk of pressure sores is higher. This is also the case if they tend to spill their bottle or their catheter bypasses or if they are over-heated and so constantly perspire.

Movement and handling

If carers are not trained in movement and handling techniques or are unable to change the individual's position without any friction or shearing occurring, the individual is at heightened risk of developing pressure sores. If the individual suffers from spasms this can cause shearing and increased pressure possibly resulting in sores.

It is vital to remember that a pressure sore can develop within a matter of hours in vulnerable individuals and can take many months to heal. It is the responsibility of the nurse to ensure that the patient's skin remains intact. This does not just mean regular changes of position while in their care (although this is important), but also ensuring appropriate pressure relieving cushions etc. are in situ when the patient leaves the ward/residential area to attend an outpatient appointment or trip out etc. This is also something that staff in transitory places such as accident and emergency or the X-ray department must remember. A wait of just a couple of hours on a hard trolley may be sufficient to cause a pressure sore. Vulnerable patients must be dealt with quickly and an awareness of pressure area care must be evident.

Family care giving

Everyone who has developed severe MS will need some help and support from others. This may be a home help visit once weekly to help with the cleaning and ironing or the individual may need 24-hour care. For most people at least some of the need for the care is met by members of their family, often their spouse or adult child. This can have profound implications for all concerned.

As with people with MS, family carers will develop their own ways of coping with the stresses and strains. Some of the most common stressors (which are listed in Table 11.2) are explored below.

Table 11.2 Common stressors for family care-givers

- Financial problems
- Lack of support from family and friends/ social isolation
- Lack of support from health and social service professionals
- Lack of sleep
- Changing roles between spouses
- Interference with social activities
- Physical strain
- Long duration of care giving*
- Caring for someone with moderate to severe MS*
- Caring for someone whose disease course is fluctuating*
- Watching a loved one become progressively disabled
- Dealing with a multitude of different professionals

* Aronson, 1997

It is known that there is a link between carers who are unsupported and higher health care costs and an increased use of emergency admissions (Anderson, 1990).

It often falls to the nurse to realise that the carer is experiencing undue strain and to offer some solutions. The carer may just need someone to talk through their fears and concerns with and the nurse can often fill this need, at least initially. However, it is important that the social worker is involved (indeed carers are now able to request an assessment from social services in their own right). The carer should be offered information and advice from the health professionals as well as the opportunity for peer support from other areas. It is known that carers who know and meet a greater number of others in similar situations to themselves are less depressed than those who know no one in similar circumstances (Pillemer and Suitor, 1996). The Carers' Association can be invaluable in this context. Carers should also be offered respite care and ultimately permanent residential care if appropriate. Respite care can take many forms. It may be that the individual with MS can attend a day-care centre once to five times a week, alternatively the family may find regular periods of residential care works better, for example, a week in a residential unit (preferably a young disabled unit if appropriate) every three months. Another option may be that social service carers can stay with the individual who has MS while the family carer spends some time away. The social worker will work with the family to find the package of care that best meets the whole family's needs.

End-stage MS

MS is not a terminal disease; the vast majority of people with MS live their normal life span and die of conditions completely unrelated to MS. It is said that people die with MS rather than of MS. However, a minority of people with severe disability can die from complications of MS. The time from disease onset to death varies widely between individuals. A survey of over 5600 people with MS extending over 45 years determined that life expectancy for people with MS is on average 11 years less than the general population (Koch-Henriksen and Brønnum-Hansen, 1999). As this is an average figure, clearly many individuals will have a normal life expectancy while others with severe disease will unfortunately die earlier than expected due to their MS. On a slightly more positive note, the same study has demonstrated that the lifespan of people with MS has in fact been steadily increasing over the last few decades. This is a greater increase than has been seen in the general population.

Cause of death can be classified in to four groups:

* complications such as pneumonia and aspiration;
* directly due to MS;
* unrelated to MS;
* suicide.

The likelihood of death occurring due to secondary complications of MS, rather than an unrelated illness, increases with increasing disability (i.e. wheelchair bound or worse) and with increasing time from onset (Weinshenker, 1997).

Death as a direct result of MS is very rare. There is an extremely rare variant type of MS known as Marburg's variant, which is often fatal within a few months of onset. This may be due to respiratory failure as a result of paralysis of the diaphragm muscles or occasionally as a result of cerebral herniation.

Suicide among people with MS has been reported to be as much as 7.5 times higher than the normal population (Sadovnick *et al.*, 1991), although another extensive study in Denmark found a twofold increase (Koch-Henriksen and Brønnum-Hansen, 1999). Whatever the actual level it is clear that the suicide rate is significantly higher among people with MS than people without MS. Specific risk factors that increase an individual's likelihood of committing suicide are listed in Table 8.1.

Causes of death unrelated to MS are similar to those of the general population, i.e. myocardial infarction, stroke and malignancy. Although the study by Sadovnick *et al.* in 1991 showed people with MS had a slightly higher risk of dying from stroke and significantly lower risk of malignancy, why this should be is not clear.

In summary the majority of people with MS can expect to live a near normal lifespan and to die of conditions unrelated to MS. A minority of people with severe and progressive MS may experience disabilities that predispose them to life-threatening complications such as pneumonia and aspiration. Suicide is also a risk, although this can be mediated by ensuring individuals receive appropriate levels of support and symptom management.

Nursing the patient with end-stage MS

End-stage MS is the phase of an individual's life when their disabilities result in severe limitations in their ability to fulfil any action and when these disabilities cause life-threatening complications that cannot be resolved. Individuals with such severe problems occurring as a result of their MS may not always have full insight into the extent of their problems and therefore prognosis. Often cognitive impairment has developed to an extent that the individual is cushioned to a large degree from their situation. However, not everyone will develop severe cognitive impairment and some individuals will be fully aware of the much shortened life span that they face.

Nursing people with end-stage MS can be draining. It is physically hard work and emotionally wearing. It rarely requires great technical skills, perhaps managing a pump feed, an air loss mattress and occasionally some oral suctioning. Nursing someone with end-stage MS, indeed anyone with severe disability resulting from MS requires us to practise the essence of our nursing skills. It is about keeping the individual comfortable and free from pain, washing the patient with care and sensitivity, preserving their privacy and dignity. It is about maintaining their skin integrity, ensuring their oral hygiene is sufficient to keep their mouths moist and clean and fresh feeling. It is about maintaining their bladder and bowel function and, most importantly, it is about respecting them as an individual.

Even if the patient cannot communicate their own needs or wishes the nurse must speak with their family and friends to learn about the patient as an individual. Has he always been clean-shaven? If so this must be maintained by nursing staff. How does she like her hair styled? Has she always hated anyone seeing her without her make-up on? The emotional support required by the patient and their family is huge. Providing this support also lies at the heart of nursing, the nurse should be there to listen (and hear what the patient and family are saying), to give everyone the chance to talk about how they are feeling. They must respect the wishes of the patient and their family and when the family's wishes may compromise the care of the patient (e.g. positioning) this must be fully explained and discussed with all concerned. The nurse must also, in conjunction with the interdisciplinary team, reassure the patient and their family that everything will be done to ensure the patient is pain free, comfortable and cared for.

As every individual with MS is different, so the way each individual and their families face dying with MS will be different. For some it will be almost a relief – an expected end to a long period of suffering. For others it will be unexpected and tragic. People will feel many different emotions such as anger, despair, relief, guilt and great sadness. Often people will feel confused – how can they be relieved that their loved one is dying, how can things have got this bad. People will feel helpless and frightened. The nurse must help the patient and their family cope with the depth of feelings experienced. Being understanding, supportive, listening, by providing continuity and ensuring the needs of the patient are met calmly, effectively and sensitively the nurse can go a long way towards helping the individuals and their family through a hugely difficult time.

Providing this level of care and support means that the nurse themselves will also require support. All nurses must be responsible for recognising this need and providing support for each other and themselves. Support should be available through a number of channels both formally, for example via supervision and/or counselling and informally from colleagues, family and friends. Each nurse must also develop their own personal strategies that enable them to relax and 'switch off' after work.

Nursing people with end-stage MS can be full of challenges (both personal and professional) and is often very difficult, but can also be immensely rewarding and satisfying and can provide us with an opportunity for growth.

CHAPTER 12

The future for people with MS

Diagnosis, treatment, symptom management and care for people with MS have come a long way in the past 10–15 years. For instance magnetic resonance imaging is now a routine diagnostic tool allowing people to be diagnosed earlier and with more certainty. Disease modifying therapies such as beta interferon and glatiramer acetate have allowed us to reduce the frequency of relapses for some people. New drugs such as tizanadine to treat spasticity and gabapentin to treat pain have found their way into the neurologist's armoury enabling better symptom management.

The importance of an interdisciplinary approach to the care of someone with MS is also now much more widely recognised. The number of MS specialist nurses has grown from four in 1995 to approximately eighty in 2001 and continues to grow. In addition the MS Society has published guidelines for the standard of care of people with MS (Freeman *et al.*, 1997), the National Institute for Clinical Excellence are also in the process of developing a similar set of guidelines. Thus, with all these recent advances, people with MS should no longer be told 'there is nothing we can do for you'.

This said there remain major gaps in our understanding of MS. For example the exact cause of MS remains unclear, the disease process itself is not fully understood and the mode of action of many existing treatments remains elusive. Research into many different aspects of MS is ongoing throughout the world and is much more prevalent now than even 15 years ago. This is due, in part at least, to interferon, which has shown that modification of MS is in fact possible and that something can be done.

Interferon has also succeeded in raising the profile of MS among researchers, health professionals and the general public alike.

A few of the many promising areas of current research are described briefly below. The future for people with MS can only get better.

Remyelination

It is well known that the disease process in MS damages the myelin of neurones in selected areas within the spinal cord and brain. It is this damage that causes delay or blocking of the conduction of impulses along the neurones which in turn results in the many different symptoms someone with MS can experience. It is also known that there is some spontaneous remyelination of damaged axons, certainly within the earlier stages of the disease. However, prolonged demyelination of individual axons will result in degeneration and loss of the axon, which subsequently results in atrophy and permanent loss of function (Trapp *et al.*, 1999).

Therefore, in theory, if axons can be remyelinated artificially then conduction of impulses along the neurones will be restored and so in turn will function. Axonal loss and therefore permanent disability should also be prevented. Research in this area is ongoing across the world and there are a number of very promising leads, however there are some fundamental problems that must first be overcome.

1. Demyelinated lesions are typically large, numerous and exist within the central nervous system where active demyelination is ongoing. If axons are to be remyelinated, a way of targeting the appropriate lesions must be found and remyelination can only be effective if used in conjunction with an agent to suppress further demyelination.
2. The correlation between lesions seen on a MR scan and the individual's function is not well understood. It is necessary to not only remyelinate lesions but also, in so doing, to restore function and this is proving more difficult (Compston *et al.*, 1996).
3. In order to enable effective remyelination, migration of the cells chosen through the central nervous system to the demyelinated lesions is essential. Survival of these cells as myelin forming cells in situ is also imperative.
4. Remyelination can only be effective if used before axonal loss occurs and therefore timing of the process is crucial and needs to be determined.
5. The most effective cells to be used for remyelination also need to be selected. Cells that have been used to date include oligodendrocyte progenitors (these have shown promise but are sourced from foetal

tissue which raises a lot of ethical questions); schwann cells (Compston *et al.*, 1996); autologous cell grafts (cells taken from the individual's central nervous system, although remyelination using these cells has yet to be demonstrated (Targett *et al.*, 1996)) and human olfactory ensheathing cells (Barnett *et al.*, 2000).

Despite these problems, work continues apace and this remains a very promising line of enquiry. It is important that people with MS are encouraged by the potential of this work but do not have their hopes raised by overlooking the obstacles still to be overcome (Scolding, 1999).

Vaccination

Without knowing the nature of the environmental factor implemented in the cause of MS, a vaccination to prevent the disease occurring at all is a long way from being a reality. However there is a lot of work ongoing to examine the feasibility of a vaccination which will protect someone diagnosed with MS from further immune mediated damage. This involves protecting the individual against the specific cells within the immune system, which trigger the process of demyelination.

Different approaches to this problem have been used; for example a T cell antigen receptor based vaccination (Bourdette *et al.*, 1994). T cells are the cells within the immune system most implicated in the pathology of demyelination. Another approach has been to use a vaccine based on the individual's own T cells which are specific for myelin basic protein (Zhang *et al.*, 1993).

This latter approach has proved the more promising of the two to date. A small study has demonstrated a reduction in relapse rate and lesion size for over half (although not all) the patients in the study (Medaer *et al.*, 1995). There is currently a phase II trial of T cell vaccination underway in America. This is as a direct result of the preliminary research cited above. (A phase II trial is one in which a moderate number of people are used and the primary outcome is to establish the safety of the medication being tested; further large-scale trials to determine effectiveness will follow if the phase II trial is successful.)

However there still remain many problems to be overcome before this can be used as an effective agent to 'switch off' MS. It is also important to remember that prevention of demyelination will only be of real benefit in patients whose MS has not progressed too far as this technique will not restore any function that has been lost.

Stem cell transplantation

Stem cells are cells that have the capacity to grow and replicate and become any cell within the human body.

The individual being treated must first donate some bone marrow, the stem cells within the bone marrow are then extracted and held outside the body. Meanwhile the individual's immune system is destroyed using radiotherapy or chemotherapy. The original stem cells are then replaced and encouraged to regenerate a new and healthy immune system.

This treatment is still very experimental and has an unacceptably high mortality rate at present (Compston, 1998b). It is currently only used at a very few centres within the USA for patients who have severe and rapidly progressing disease.

While none of these treatments is currently at the stage where we can use them in clinical practice, they serve to illustrate a fraction of the research that is currently being undertaken in MS. This research is not restricted to finding a way of suppressing the disease, there is also a lot of work being undertaken to elicit the pathophysiology, aetiology and natural history of MS. Indeed both types of research must proceed hand in hand as one informs the other.

Research is also ongoing into symptom management. For example the cannabis study which is underway in the UK at the time of writing; it is hoped that this study will demonstrate the effectiveness of cannabis as an anti-spasticity medication. In America a new treatment for daytime sleepiness, modafinil, has been licensed for use in narcolepsy. This has been shown to be effective in reducing daytime fatigue without affecting the quality of night-time sleep (US Modafinil in Narcolepsy Study Group, 2000). A study of 72 people with MS using modafinil showed that it was effective in reducing fatigue at a dose of 200mg daily but was not effective at a dose of 400mg daily. It was also shown to be most effective in people with relapsing-remitting MS (Rammohan *et al.*, 2000). Further research is needed to establish the reason for the dose effect and also to repeat the study using larger numbers of people with MS. It will also be important to compare the effectiveness of modafinil with existing agents such as amantadine.

It is not just neurologists who are forging ahead in research, other members of the interdisciplinary team are also undertaking research projects to identify best practice in their care of people with MS. This includes validation of therapies that we 'know' work but have never been proven, e.g. physiotherapy (Wiles *et al.*, 2001) and the role of the MS specialist nurse (work ongoing). Rehabilitation itself is another area that is the subject of much review and research (e.g. Freeman *et al.*, 1999). Unanswered questions within rehabilitation include:

- How long do patients retain the improvements noted during inpatient rehabilitation once they have been discharged?
- Which aspects of rehabilitation are the most effective?
- How cost effective is rehabilitation?
- What impact does rehabilitation have on quality of life (Freeman and Thompson, 1997)?

Studies looking at different aspects of rehabilitation are currently underway across the world and it is hoped that some of these questions will be addressed by the outcomes of these studies.

This overview of current research in MS hopefully provides an inkling of the scope and scale that research into all areas of MS has now achieved. It is hoped that this growth in interest and subsequently understanding of the different aspects of MS continues. People with MS and health professionals working with them should be encouraged that slowly but surely the pieces of the jigsaw that is MS will be found and slotted into place, so, in time, improving life enormously for anyone touched by MS.

Resources

Advice on benefits

Benefit Enquiry line
0800 882200
(Northern Ireland 0800 220674)

Part of the benefits agency, can supply application forms and answer general enquiries.

National Association of Citizens' Advice Bureaux
Myddleton House
115–123 Pentonville Road
London N1 9LZ
020 7833 2181

Citizens' Advice Bureaux also provide advice and information on a wide range of other topics

Carers Information

Carers National Association
Ruth Pitter House
20–25 Glasshouse Yard
London EC1A 4JT
020 7490 8818
Helpline: 0808 808 777

The Carers Association produce a wide range of information for carers as well as running a helpline and providing advice and support for carers.

Complementary Therapies

British Complementary Medicine Association
249 Fosse Road South
Leicester LE3 1AE
0116 282 5511

Deals with registration of a wide range of complementary practitioners.

Council for Complementary and Alternative Medicine
63 Jeddo Road
London W12 6HQ
020 8735 0632

Deals with registration of acupuncture, herbal medicine, homeopathy and osteopathy.

Continence

Continence Foundation
307 Hatton Square
16 Baldwins Gardens
London EC1N 7RJ
Helpline: 020 7831 9831

Helpline run by nurse specialists. They can offer advice to patients and health professionals and have a range of information leaflets available.

Counselling

British Association for Counselling
1 Regent Place
Rugby
Warwickshire
CV21 2PJ
0870 443 5252
www.counselling.co.uk

CRUSE (Bereavement) Head Office
126 Sheen Road
Richmond
Surrey TW9 1UR
020 8940 4818

Disability rights

Disability Rights Commission
Freepost M1D 02164
Stratford upon Avon
CV37 9BR
08457 622633
www.drc-gb.org

They can provide a range of information pertaining to the rights of
people with disabilities.

RADAR (Royal Association for Disability and Rehabilitation)
12 City Forum
250 City Road
London EC1V 8AF
020 7250 3222

They are an information and campaigning organisation. They can also
provide a key for use in disabled toilets around the UK for a nominal fee.

Driving

Disabled Drivers Association
National Headquarters
Ashwellthorpe
Norwich NR16 1EX
01508 489449

Provide information and advice on a range of mobility issues for people
with disabilities. They also produce a newsletter for members with information about concessions, products and events. A Technical Officer is
available who can offer advice on specific issues.

Motability
Goodman House
Station Approach
Harlow
Essex CM20 2ET
01279 635666

Employment

Employment Opportunities for People with Disabilities
123 Minories
London EC3N 1NT
020 7481 2727

16 offices around the UK. They provide support and advice on a wide range of issues connected with employment for people with disabilities.

Rehab UK
Brain Injury Vocational Services
Windermere House
Kendal Avenue
London W3 0XA
020 8896 2333

A number of regional offices. They can provide assessments at home or at work and make recommendations about equipment and adaptations that may be needed. They also provide advice, support and training for people with disabilities trying to return to work.

Government departments

Department of Health
Richmond House
79 Whitehall
London SW1A 2NS
020 7210 4850
www.doh.gov.uk

NICE (National Institute for Clinical Excellence)
11 Strand
London WC2N 5HR
020 7766 9191
www.nice.org.uk

MS specific charities

Multiple Sclerosis Society
National MS Centre
372 Edgware Road
London NW2 6ND
020 8438 0701
Helpline: 0808 800 8000
www.mssociety.org.uk

Multiple Sclerosis Society Scotland
Rural Centre
Hallyards Road
Ingliston
Edinburgh
EH28 8NZ
0131 472 4106

Multiple Sclerosis Society Northern Ireland
34 Annadale Road
Belfast BT7 3JJ
028 90802802

The MS Society produce a wide range of information leaflets free of charge and produce a bimonthly magazine for members. They have many local branches providing a range of services and support to people with MS and their families. The MS Society also fund research and campaign for improved services for people with MS.

Multiple Sclerosis (Research) Charitable Trust (MSRCT)
Spirella Building
Bridge Road
Letchworth
Herts SG6 4ET
01462 476700
www.msresearchtrust.org.uk

The MSRCT produce information packs for both people with MS and for health professionals; they also provide comprehensive library services for health professionals working with people with MS. The MS Nurse Forum is run by the MSRCT and as part of the support and information offered to health professionals, they organise a number of study days and conferences throughout the year. They are also involved in campaigning for better services for people with MS across the UK and fund various research projects.

Association of MS Therapy Centres
Unit 1 Saxbane Crescent
Howe Moss Crescent
Kirkhill Industrial Estate
Dyce
Aberdeen AB2 0GN
01224 771105

Federation of MS Therapy Centres
Bradbury House
155 Barkers Lane
Bedford MK41 9RX
01234 325781
www.ms-selfhelp.org

Therapy centres provide access to hyberbaric oxygen and a number of other complementary therapies. They also provide a meeting place for people with MS to gain support and advice. They publish a bimonthly magazine about living with MS.

International Federation of MS Centres (IFMSS)
www.ifmss.org.uk

This is a very informative web site with links to many other sites and journals.

Nursing

Royal College of Nursing
RCN Headquarters
20 Cavendish Square
London W1M 0DB
020 7409 3333

Library and information services: 020 7647 3610
www.rcn.org.uk

International Organisation of MS Nurses (IOMSN)
PO Box 450
Teaneck
New Jersey 07666
USA
www.iomsn.org

Sexuality and parenting

Disability, Pregnancy and Parenthood International
The National Centre for Disabled Parents
Unit F9 Fonthill Road
London N4 3JH
0800 018 4730

Run by disabled parents to promote awareness and support for disabled people during pregnancy and throughout parenthood. They work with parents and health and social work professionals and publish a quarterly journal.

Impotence Association
PO Box 10296
London SW7 9WH
020 8767 7791

They provide free information and advice on treatments for both men and women with sexual dysfunction.

SPOD (Association to aid the sexual and personal relationships of people with a disability)
286 Camden Road
London N7 0BJ
020 7607 8851

SPOD is a client led organisation, which promotes disabled people's rights to equal access to advice, education and treatment in all areas of sexual and personal relationships. They produce a range of information leaflets and run a helpline which can be accessed both by clients and health professionals needing advice on how to manage a particular problem.

APPENDIX II

Glossary

Astrocytes These are highly branched cells which are an integral part of the blood–brain barrier and which also serve to support neurones.

Ataxia This is usually applied to the way in which an individual walks, but can also be applied to arm movements. It refers to movements that are uncoordinated. People who have an ataxic gait tend to walk with their feet more widely apart as this wide-base gives them a little more stability.

Axonal loss If the same axons within the central nervous system are constantly attacked and myelin is removed, they will eventually cease to remyelinate. Once the axon is left denuded, or if there are no longer any neuroglial cells in the vicinity, the axon itself is destroyed and so axonal loss occurs. It is thought to be this phenomenon which is largely responsible for the permanent loss of function that can result from MS.

B Lymphocytes Particular cells within the immune system which produce antibodies (responsible for producing antibodies which bind with myelin in people who have MS).

Babinski reflex The lateral aspect of the sole of an individual's foot is stroked firmly with a blunt pointer from the heel to the ball of the foot. If the toes curl downward (i.e. down-going plantars) this is normal, if the toes curl upward (i.e. up-going plantars) an abnormality of the pyramidal tract is indicated.

Blood–brain barrier (BBB) Foot like processes of astrocytes surround the endothelial cells of the blood vessels within the central nervous system. This forms a barrier against unwanted cells and molecules passing from the blood stream and into the central nervous system.

Cerebellum An area at the rear of the brain which controls balance, coordination and skilled movements.

CNS This stands for central nervous system which comprises the brain and spinal cord, demyelination occurs only within the CNS in people with MS.

Diplopia This means double vision, which is quite a common symptom in MS and tends to resolve spontaneously. Wearing a patch over one eye when reading, watching television etc. can help.

Disease modifying therapies These are treatments that can be given to some individuals with MS to alter the course of their MS. This group includes the beta interferons, glatiramer acetate and others such as immunoglobulins and mitoxantrone.

Dysarthria This is a mechanical difficulty in speaking, i.e. the muscles of mouth and tongue are unable to function efficiently to produce the sounds needed to vocalise effectively.

Dysphagia This is difficulty swallowing. The first signs of a problem in people with MS are often that they cough and splutter when drinking.

Dysphasia Difficulty processing speech. In MS this usually presents as a problem with word finding (i.e. expressive dysphasia).

EDSS The Expanded Disability Status Scale is a tool used to measure disability in MS.

Epidemiology This is the study of the pattern of a disease, e.g. where, when and in whom does it occur?

Euphoria An emotional state caused by MS. People with euphoria respond to their disease and its attendant difficulties with inappropriate good humour. This is a direct result of demyelination but is not normally treated as it generally makes everything much easier to cope with for patient, family and staff alike.

Fatigue Fatigue can be one of the most difficult symptoms to cope with. The individual feels drained and the tiredness experienced is out of all proportion to any activity undertaken. It is often very difficult for family and friends to appreciate how limiting fatigue can be.

Foot drop The individual with foot drop is unable to fully dorsi-flex (i.e. bend upwards) their foot when walking, this in turn leads to trips and stumbles. It can be corrected with a foot splint, which holds the foot in a more normal position.

Frequency This is an epidemiological term, which asks how often does the disease occur? This is worked out by dividing the number of people who develop the disease in a given area within a year (the incidence) with the number of people in the general population who are at risk of developing the same disease in the same area within the same time period.

Gadolinium This is a contrast agent used in MRI scanning. The patient is injected with a gadolinium compound and the scan is taken. It is then possible to identify on the scan any breaches in the blood–brain barrier, which represent areas of active disease.

Glial cell These are the cells within the central nervous system which are responsible for physically supporting neurones.

Grey matter This is the part of the central nervous system which consists of cell bodies (as opposed to axons).

IDT Interdisciplinary team, in order to meet the needs of someone with MS a team of health professionals from many different disciplines must work together as a well-knit team.

Ig G index Immunoglobulin G is a protein which is usually present in the cerebrospinal fluid of people experiencing demyelination. The Ig G index is a comparison of the amount of Ig G in the CSF with the amount in the individual's plasma. People with MS usually have an Ig G index of at least 0.7.

Incidence This is an epidemiological term and represents the number of people who develop a particular disease in a given area in one year.

Interneurones Neurones which reside entirely within the central nervous system.

Intravenous methyl prednisolone (IVMP) This is an intravenous steroid which is sometimes given to treat an acute relapse of MS. High doses are given over 3–5 days, usually with good effect.

L'Hermittes sign This occurs fairly commonly in people with MS. When they bend their head forwards, they experience a feeling like an electric shock down their neck and back.

Lymphocytes These are cells found within the blood and lymph system, which form part of the immune system.

Magnetic resonance imaging (MRI) This is a type of scan which can be used to look at any part of the body. In the context of MS it is used primarily as a diagnostic or research tool to examine the central nervous system. The patient is placed inside the scanner (effectively a large magnet), a radio wave is sent in and subsequently turned off, the signal then emitted by the patient is interpreted to form the MRI scans with which we are familiar.

Marburg's MS This is an extremely rare variant of MS in which the individual becomes profoundly disabled very quickly, often within a matter of months. It is effectively terminal.

Methyl prednisolone A steroid given over 3–5 days either intravenously or orally, to treat an acute relapse of MS. Methyl prednisolone makes no difference to the long-term prognosis but can help reduce the short-term impact of a relapse.

Microglia These cells migrate to the site of injury within the central nervous system and phagocytise debris, they are known to be involved in the inflammatory process which occurs in MS and to facilitate loss of myelin.

Myelin This is a fatty substance which surrounds axons. It acts as insulation and facilitates the conduction of impulses along the axon. The thicker the myelin, the quicker the impulse can be transmitted. It is myelin that is destroyed by the immune response in MS.

Neuroglia These are the cells found within the central nervous system which act as supporting cells for the neurones (it literally means 'nerve glue').

Nodes of Ranvier These are the gaps in the myelin along the length of the axon. The impulses being transmitted along the axon can jump between the gaps so facilitating conduction. The frequency of the nodes determines the speed of transmission of impulses along the axon.

Oligoclonal bands These illustrate the presence of immunoglobulin G. In someone with MS they are usually present in the CSF but not the blood plasma.

Oligodendrocytes These are the cells in the central nervous system that are responsible for myelinating axons. Each oligodendrocyte is capable of myelinating many different axons by wrapping its cell process around the axon in a spiral manner.

Optic neuritis This is often one of the presenting signs of MS (although not everyone with optic neuritis will go on to develop MS). The optic nerve becomes inflamed; this causes pain behind the eye and often results in blurred vision.

Paresis Weakness, usually in an affected limb or limbs e.g. hemi-paresis which means one side (or half) of the individual is weak.

Parasthesia A sensation of pins and needles.

Periventricular tracts These are bundles of axons within the cerebrum that form the roof of the ventricles within the brain. They consist of bundles of axons responsible for transferring impulses from one part of the brain to another. They are particularly prone to developing plaques of demyelination.

Plaques These are the areas within the central nervous system where the myelin has been destroyed. On a magnetic resonance scan they usually show up as small white areas.

Prevalence This is an epidemiological term and indicates the number of people who have a particular disease in a given area at a given point in time.

Primary progressive MS Approximately 10% of people with MS have primary progressive disease. They tend to deteriorate from onset of the disease and their rate of deterioration can be rapid (though is not always).

Primary symptoms These are symptoms occurring directly as a result of demyelination.

Proprioception This describes position sense, e.g. the way that we know without looking where our feet are. This sense can be adversely affected in people with MS.

Relapse The development of new symptoms or the recurrence of old symptoms that last at least 48 hours.

Relapsing progressive MS Individuals follow a progressive course with relapses superimposed on top.

Relapsing-remitting MS People with this type of MS follow a course consisting of periods of fairly acute deterioration followed by a full or partial recovery of function.

Remission A full or partial improvement in symptoms and function. Thought to be due to partial remyelination within the central nervous system.

Remyelination The myelin of an axon is damaged during a period of acute inflammation (i.e. a relapse), once the inflammation settles down it is thought that there can be some subsequent repair of the myelin by remaining oligodendrocytes. This accounts, at least in part, for the period of recovery (i.e. remission) which usually follows a relapse.

Romberg's test The patient is asked to stand erect with their eyes shut, if they lose their balance it is said to be a positive result and implies damage to the dorsal column.

Secondary progressive MS People with this type of MS have progressed beyond relapsing-remitting disease and are now following a deteriorating course. The speed at which an individual is likely to deteriorate varies hugely and some may well remain fairly stable.

Secondary symptoms These occur as a result of complications of primary symptoms, e.g. recurrent urine infections due to incomplete emptying of the bladder.

Silent plaques (shadow plaques) These are plaques, which can be seen on a MRI scan, but which produce no clinical signs. They often indicate areas of remyelination.

Spasticity This is defined as an increased resistance to passive movement. People generally feel stiff and may have difficulty walking.

T Lymphocytes Particular cells within the immune system, which destroy antibody-antigen complexes. In MS they destroy the myelin–antibody complex formed when the B lymphocytes produce antibodies that bind with the myelin.

Tertiary symptoms The psychosocial consequences of living with primary and secondary symptoms of MS, e.g. low self-esteem, unemployment and role changes.

Transition phase This is the phase when an individual's MS is changing from relapsing-remitting to secondary progressive. It can last several months to a couple of years and can be a difficult time for all concerned.

White matter This is the part of the central nervous system, which consists of axons, and is therefore the area most affected by demyelination.

References

ABN (2001) Guidelines for the use of Beta interferon's and glatiramer acetate in multiple sclerosis. London: Association of British Neurologists.

Achiron A, Gabbay U, Gilad R, Hassain-Baer S et al. (1998) Intravenous immunoglobulin treatment in MS: effect on relapses, Neurology 50: 398–402.

Alusi SH, Glickman S, Aziz TZ, Bain PG (1999) Editorial: Tremor in multiple sclerosis, Journal of Neurology, Neurosurgery and Psychiatry 66: 131–4.

Amato MP, Ponziani G (1999) Quantification of impairment in MS: discussion of the scales in use, Multiple Sclerosis 5(4): 216–19.

Anderson JM (1990) Home care management in chronic illness and the self-care movement: an analysis of ideologies and economic processes influencing policy decisions, Advanced Nursing Science 12: 71–83.

Andersson M, Alvarez-Cermeno J, Bernardi G, Cogato I et al. (1994) Cerebrospinal fluid in the diagnosis of MS: a consensus report, Journal of Neurology, Neurosurgery and Psychiatry 57: 897–902.

Annoni JM, Vuagnat H, Frischknecht R, Vebelhart D (1998) Percutaneous endoscopic gastrostomy in neurological rehabilitation: a report of six cases, Disability & Rehabilitation 20(8): 308–14.

Anon (1976) The P-LI-SS-IT model: a proposed conceptual scheme for behavioural treatment of sexual problems, Journal of Sex Education Therapy 2: 1–15.

Antonak RF, Livneh H (1995) Psychosocial adaptation to disability and its investigation among persons with MS, Social Science Medicine 40(8): 1099-1118.

Arnason BGW (1993) Interferon beta in multiple sclerosis, Neurology 43: 641–3.

Arnason BG, Dianzani F (1998) Correlation of the appearance of anti-interferon antibodies during treatment and diminution of efficacy: summary of an international workshop on anti-interferon antibodies, Journal of Cytokine Research 18: 639–44.

Aronson KJ (1997) Quality of life among persons with multiple sclerosis and their care givers, Neurology 48: 74–80.

Avorn J, Monane M, Gurwitz H, Glynn RJ et al. (1994) Reduction of bacteruria and pyuria after ingestion of cranberry juice, JAMA 271: 751–4.

Bain L (1996) Neurodegenerative diseases: sustaining hope, Professional Nurse 11(10): 659–61.

Barnes M (1999) Modern management & spasticity: using a combined approach, Progress in Neurology and Psychiatry, May/June.

Barnes M (2000a) Management of spasticity – pharmacological agents. In CP Hawkins, JS Wolinsky (eds), Principles of Treatments in Multiple Sclerosis. Oxford: Butterworth-Heinemann.

Barnes M (2000b) Treatment of acute relapse. Chapter 2 in CP Hawkins, JS Wolinsky (eds), Principles of Treatments in Multiple Sclerosis. Oxford: Butterworth-Heinemann.

Barnes D, Hughes RAC, Morris RW, Wade-Jones O et al. (1997) Randomised trial of oral and intravenous methylprednisolone in acute relapses of multiple sclerosis, Lancet 349: 902–6.

Barnes M, Thompson A, Bates D and the panel members (1999) Basics of Best Practice in the Management of Multiple Sclerosis. MS Society and MS Research Trust.

Barnett SC, Alexander CL, Iwashita Y, Gilson JM et al. (2000) Identification of a human olfactory ensheathing cell that can effect transplant-mediated remyelination of demyelinated central nervous system axons, Brain 123(8): 1581–8.

Bates D, Barkhof F, Clanet M and members of the MS Forum Workshop (1993) The diagnosis of multiple sclerosis. Proceedings of the MS Forum Modern Management Workshop. Professional Postgraduate Services Ltd.

Bates D, Ebers G, Fieschi C, Lucas K et al. (1999) MS Forum: Clinicians and People with Multiple Sclerosis – Views on Multiple Sclerosis and Its Management. Worthing: PPS Europe.

Beck RW, Cleary PA, Anderson PAC Jr (1992) A randomised controlled trial of corticosteroids in the treatment of acute optic neuritis, New England Journal of Medicine 326: 581–8.

Benson GS (1997) Sexual dysfunction in the patient with multiple sclerosis. In CS Raine, HF McFarland, WW Tourtellotte (eds), Multiple Sclerosis. London: Chapman & Hall, p. 379.

Binnie A, Titchen A (1999) Freedom to practice. In J Lathlean (ed.), The Development of Patient-Centred Nursing. Oxford: Butterworth-Heinemann.

Bitsch A, Wegener C, da Costa C, Bunkowski S et al. (1999) Lesion development in Marburg's type of acute multiple sclerosis: from inflammation to demyelination, Multiple Sclerosis 5(3): 138–46.

Borràs C, Rio J, Porcel J, Barrios M et al. (1999) Emotional state of patients with relapsing remitting MS treated with beta interferon 1b, Neurology 52: 1636–9.

Bourdette DN, Whitham RH, Chou YK, Morrison WJ et al. (1994) Immunity to T cell receptor peptides in multiple sclerosis. I. Successful immunisation of patients with synthetic V beta 5.2 and V beta 6.1 CDR2 peptides, Journal of Immunology 152: 2510–19.

Brechin M, Burgess M (2001) Designing an education tool for patients with multiple sclerosis, Professional Nurse 16(11): 1471–4.

British National Formulary (1999) BMA Pharmaceutical Society of Great Britain, March.

Brønnum-Hansen H, Koch-Henriksen N, Hyllested K (1994) Survival of patients with multiple sclerosis in Denmark: a nation-wide, long term epidemiological survey, Neurology 44: 1901–7.

Burgess M (1998) Patient's views of interferon therapy in MS, Professional Nurse 13(9).

Burgess M (n.d.) unpublished data on file.

Burnfield A (1982) Psychosocial aspects of MS, Physiotherapy 68(5): 149–50.

Cajal SR (1913) Contribucion al conocmiento de la neuroglia del cerebra humano, Trabajos del Laboratorio de Investigaciones Biologicas 11: 255–315.

Carruthers A (1992) A force to promote bonding and well being, therapeutic touch and massage, Professional Nurse, Feb.: 297–300.

Carswell R (1838) Pathological Anatomy: Illustrations of the Elementary Forms of Disease. London: Orme, Brown, Green & Longman.

Castledine G (2000) Hope: a key concept in the psychology of nursing, British Journal of Nursing 9(14): 954.

Chandler BJ, Brown S (1998) Sex and relationship dysfunction in neurological disability, Journal of Neurology, Neurosurgery and Psychiatry 65: 877–80.

Clanet M, Arnason B, Borgel F, Fowler C et al. (1994) The symptoms of multiple sclerosis and their management. Proceedings of the MS Forum Modern Management Workshop, Paris. Worthing: PPS Services Europe Ltd.

Clark CC (1986) Wellness Nursing. New York: Springer.

Clifford DB (1983) Tetrahydrocanibinol for tremor in multiple sclerosis, Annals of Neurology 13: 669–71.

Cohen RA, Fisher M (1989) Amantadine treatment of fatigue associated with MS, Archives of Neurology 46: 676–80.

Collins Paperback English Dictionary (1990) 2nd edn. London and Glasgow: Collins.

Comi G, Filippi M for the Copaxone MRI Study Group (1999) The effect of glatiramer acetate (Copaxone) on disease activity as measured by cerebral MRI in patients with relapsing-remitting MS (RRMS): a multi-center, randomised, double-blind placebo controlled study extended by open-label treatment, Neurology 52(S2): A289.

Compston A (1998a) Distribution of multiple sclerosis. In A Compston, G Ebers, H Lassman, I McDonald et al. (eds), McAlpines Multiple Sclerosis, 3rd edn. London: Churchill Livingstone.

Compston A (1998b) Future prospects. In A Compston, G Ebers, H Lassman, I McDonald et al. (eds), McAlpines Multiple Sclerosis, 3rd edn, Chapter 14. London: Churchill Livingstone.

Compston A (1998c) The story of multiple sclerosis. In A Compston, G Ebers, H Lassman, I McDonald et al. (eds), McAlpines Multiple Sclerosis, 3rd edn. London: Churchill Livingstone.

Compston A (1998d) Treatment and management of multiple sclerosis. In A Compston, G Ebers, H Lassman, I McDonald et al. (eds), McAlpines Multiple Sclerosis, 3rd edn, Chapter 14. London: Churchill Livingstone.

Compston A, Lucas K and participants of MS Forum workshop (1996) Biosynthesis of Myelin: Consequences for Remyelination Strategies, pp. 26–8. Worthing: PPS Europe Ltd.

Compston DAS, Evans CD, Feneley RCL, McLellan DL et al. (1993) Working Party Report on Multiple Sclerosis. London: British Society of Rehabilitation Medicine.

Confavreux C, Hutchinson M, Hours MM, Cortinovis-Tourniaire P et al. (1998) Rate of pregnancy related relapse in multiple sclerosis, The New England Journal of Medicine 339(5): 285–91.

Conference Report (1999) Management of neurodegenerative disorders, Hospital Medicine 60(7), July.

Conference Report (2000) Neurodegenerative disorders: a team approach, British Journal of Therapy and Rehabilitation 7(2).

Crenshaw TL, Goldberg JP (1996) Sexual dysfunction in multiple sclerosis, Archives of Physical Medical Rehabilitation 65: 125–8.

Crossman AR, Neary D (1998) Neuroanatomy: An Illustrated Colour Text. London: Churchill Livingstone.

Cullis PA, O'Brien CF, Truong DD, Koller M et al. (1998) Botulinum toxin type B: an open label, dose escalation, safety and preliminary efficacy study in cervical dystonia patients, Advanced Neurology 78: 227–30.

Davis E, Barnes M (2000) Botulinum toxin and spasticity, Journal of Neurology, Neurosurgery and Psychiatry 69: 143–9.

Dean G, Elian M (1997) Age at immigration to England of Asian and Caribbean immigrants and the risk of developing multiple sclerosis, Journal of Neurology, Neurosurgery and Psychiatry 63: 565–8.

Department of Health (1999) A First Class Service: Quality in the New NHS.

DFEE (1995) The Disability Discrimination Act 1995. A Guide for Everybody. DL160 Revised Edition.

Doherty W, Winder A (2000) Indwelling catheters: practical guidelines for catheter blockage, British Journal of Nursing 9(18): 2006–14.

Dworkin RH, Bates D, Millar JHD, Paty DW (1984) Linoleic acid and multiple sclerosis: a reanalysis of three double-blind trials, Neurology 34: 1441–5.

Dyer O (2001) Cannabis trial launched in patients with MS, BMJ 322: 192.

Eardley I, Sethia K (1998a) Intracorporeal injection therapy. In Erectile Dysfunction. Mosby International, p. 79.

Eardley I, Sethia K (1998b) Neurological disease. In Erectile Dysfunction. Mosby International, p. 3.

Eardley I, Sethia K (1998c) Non-invasive therapy for erectile dysfunction. In Erectile Dysfunction. Mosby International, p. 75.

Ebers GC, Paty DW (1998) Natural history studies and applications to clinical trials. Chapter 6 in DW Paty, GC Ebers (eds), Multiple Sclerosis. Contemporary Neurology Series. Philadelphia: FA Davies Co.

Ebers GC, Arnason B, Bates D and MS Forum Workshop Participants (1998) Environmental factors in multiple sclerosis. Proceedings of the MS Forum Modern Management Workshop, Montreal, Canada, 1999. Worthing: PPS Europe.

Eckford S, Swami K, Jackson S, Abrams PH (1994) Desmopressin in the treatment of nocturia and enuresis in patients with multiple sclerosis, British Journal of Urology 74: 733–5.

European Study Group on interferon beta 1b in secondary progressive MS (1998). Placebo controlled, multi-centre, randomised trial of interferon beta 1b in the treatment of secondary progressive MS. Lancet 352: 1491–7.

Fatigue Guidelines Development Panel members (1998) Fatigue and Multiple Sclerosis. Evidence Based Management Strategies for Fatigue in Multiple Sclerosis. Multiple Sclerosis Council for Clinical Practice Guidelines. Paralysed Veterans of America.

Fazekas F, Strasser-Fuchs, Sorensen PS (1999) Intravenous immunoglobulin trials in multiple sclerosis, International Multiple Sclerosis Journal 6(1): 15–21.

Fazekas F, Deisenhammer F, Strasser-Fuchs S, Nahler et al. (1997) Randomised placebo-controlled trial of monthly intravenous immunoglobulin therapy in relapsing-remitting MS, Lancet 349: 589–93.

Feinstein A (1995) Multiple sclerosis and depression: an etiologic conundrum, Canadian Journal of Psychiatry 40: 573–6.

Feinstein A (1999) MS and pathological laughing and crying. Chapter 4 in The Clinical Neuropsychiatry of Multiple Sclerosis. Cambridge: Cambridge University Press.

Feinstein A (2000) Neurobehavioral abnormalities. Chapter 16 in CP Hawkins, JS Wolinsky (eds), Principles of Treatments in Multiple Sclerosis. Oxford: Butterworth-Heinemann.

Few C (1993) Safer Sex. Community Outlook, 7 Sept, 13–18.

Fieschi C (1999) Shock of MS under-estimated by many physicians, Medical Express Reports 11(4). www.cambridge-medical.com

Foley FW, Sanders A (1997a) Sexuality, multiple sclerosis and women, MS Management 4(1).

Foote AW, Piaza D, Holcombe J, Paul P et al. (1990) Hope: self-esteem and social support in persons with multiple sclerosis, Journal of Neuroscience Nursing 22(3): 155–9.

Forbes RB, Lees A, Waugh N, Swingler RJ (1999) Population based cost utility study of beta interferon 1b in secondary progressive multiple sclerosis, BMJ 319: 1529–33.

Forbes SB (1994) Hope: an essential need in the elderly, Journal of Gerontological Nursing 20(6): 5–10.

Ford HL, Johnson MH (1995) Telling your patient he/she has multiple sclerosis, Postgraduate Medical Journal 71: 449–52.

Fowler CJ (1996) Investigation of the neurogenic bladder, Journal of Neurology, Neurosurgery and Psychiatry 60(6): 6–13.

Fox JP (1970) Epidemiology, Man and Disease. Toronto: Macmillan.

Frederikson S, Kam-Hansen S (1989) The 150 year anniversary of multiple sclerosis: does its early history give an etiological clue?, Perspectives in Biology and Medicine 32(2): 237–43.

Frederikson S, Arnason B, Bates D and members of the MS Forum workshop (1996) Design and Interpretation of Clinical Trials in Multiple Sclerosis. MS Forum Proceedings of the MS Forum Modern Management Workshop. Stockholm: PPS Europe Ltd.

Freeman JA, Thompson AJ (1997) Is inpatient rehabilitation effective in multiple sclerosis? Chapter 23 in AJ Thompson, C Polman, R Hohlfeld (eds), Multiple Sclerosis: Clinical Challenges and Controversies. London: Martin Dunitz.

Freeman JA, Langdon DW, Hobart JC, Thompson AJ (1999) Inpatient rehabilitation in multiple sclerosis: do the benefits carry over into the community?, Neurology 52: 50–6.

Freeman JA, Johnson J, Rollinson S, Thompson AJ et al. (1997) Standards of Healthcare for people with MS. MS Society of Great Britain and Northern Ireland and Neurorehabilitation and Therapy Services Directorate of the National Hospital for Neurology and Neurosurgery.

Frost J (1992) Herbalism: An overview of an ancient art. Origins and development of herbal therapies, Professional Nurse, Jan.: 237–41.

Goldberg P (1974) Multiple sclerosis: Vitamin D and calcium as environmental determinants of prevalence (A viewpoint). Part I: Sunlight, dietary factors and epidemiology, International Journal of Environmental Studies 6: 19–27.

Goodin DS, Ebers GC, Johnson KP, Rodriguez M et al. (1999) The relationship of MS to physical trauma and psychological stress, Neurology 52: 1737–45.

Gopee N (2000) Self-assessment and the concept of the lifelong learning nurse, British Journal of Nursing 9(11): 724–9.

Halliday AM, McDonald WI, Mushlin J (1973) Visual evoked responses in diagnosing multiple sclerosis, British Medical Journal 4: 661–4.

Hawkins CP, Wolinsky JS (eds) (2000) Principles of Treatments in Multiple Sclerosis. Chapter 5. Oxford: Butterworth-Heinemann.

Hawksey B, Williams J (2000) Rehabilitation: the role of the nurse. A workbook. London: RCN.

Hegevary ST (1982) The Change to Primary Nursing. St Louis: C V Mosby.

Henderson V (1966) The Nature of Nursing. London: Collier Macmillan.

Hernandez-Reif M, Field T, Fielt T, Theakston H (1998) Multiple sclerosis patients benefit from massage therapy, Journal of Bodywork and Movement Therapy 2(3): 168–74.

Herndon RM (2000) Treatment of multiple sclerosis with the beta interferons. Comparative risks and benefits. In A Wagstaff (ed.), Drug Treatment of Multiple Sclerosis. Adis International.

Herndon RM, Rudick RA (1983) Multiple sclerosis: the spectrum of severity, Archives of Neurology 40: 531–2.

Hickey JV (1997) The Clinical Practice of Neurological and Neurosurgical Nursing, 4th edn. Philadelphia: JB Lippincott.

Hohlfeld H (1999) Immunological basis for the therapy of multiple sclerosis, Acta Neurol. Belg. 99: 40–3.

Holland N, Halper J (1999) Primary care management of multiple sclerosis, ADVANCE for Nurse Practitioners, March, 1–8.

Holmgren E, Giuliano F, Hulting C et al. (1998) cited in Chapter 8, I Eardley, K Sethia, Erectile Dysfunction. Mosby International.

Hoverd PA, Fowler CJ (1998) Desmopressin in the treatment of daytime urinary frequency in patients with multiple sclerosis, Journal of Neurology, Neurosurgery and Psychiatry 65: 778–80.

Hunt GM, Oakeshott P, Whittaker RH (1996) Intermittent catheterisation: simple, safe and effective, but underused, BMJ 312: 103–7.

Huntley A, Ernst E (2000) Complementary and alternative therapies for treating multiple sclerosis symptoms: a systematic review, Complementary Therapies in Medicine 8: 97–105.

Husted C, Pham L, Hekking A, Niederman R (1999) Improving quality of life for people with chronic conditions: the example of T'ai chi and multiple sclerosis, Alternative Therapies 5(5): 70–4.

Hutchins JB, Naftel JP, Ard MD (1997) The cell biology of neurones and glia. In DE Haines (ed.), Fundamental Neuroscience. London: Churchill Livingstone.

INFB Multiple Sclerosis Study Group (1993) Interferon-beta 1b is effective in relapsing-remitting multiple sclerosis. I Clinical results of a multi-centre, randomised, double blind, placebo controlled trial, Neurology 43: 655–61.

Iverson LL (2000) The Science of Marijuana. Oxford: Oxford University Press.

Jacobs DJ, Cookfair DL, Rudick RA, Herndon RM et al. (1996) Intramuscular beta interferon 1a for disease progression in relapsing multiple sclerosis, Annals of Neurology 39: 285–94.

Johnson KP, Brookes BR, Cohen JA, Ford CC et al. (1995) Copolymer 1 reduces relapse rate and improves disability in relapsing-remitting multiple sclerosis: results of a phase III multi-centre, double blind, placebo controlled trial, Neurology 45: 1268–76.

Junemann KP, Manning M, Krautschick A, Alken P (1996) 15 years of injection therapy in erectile dysfunction – a review, International Journal of Impotence Research 8: A60.

Kalb RC (2000) Psychosocial issues in secondary progressive MS: a unique set of challenges, International Journal of MS Care (supplement based on the annual meeting of the Consortium of MS Centres), 22 June.

Kalb RC, LaRocca NG (1997) Sexuality and family planning. In J Halper, N Holland (eds), Comprehensive Nursing Care in Multiple Sclerosis. New York: Demos Vermande.

Kamansek J (1999) Continuous intrathecal baclofen infusions: an introduction and overview, Axon, June, 93–8.

Keen J (2000) What's up, Doc? MS Matters 30: 12. MS Society of Great Britain and Northern Ireland.

Kleijnen J, Knipschield P (1995) Hyberbaric oxygen for multiple sclerosis: review of controlled trials, Acta Neurologica Scandinavia 91: 330–4.

Koch-Herriksen N, Brønnum-Hansen H (1999) Survival in multiple sclerosis. Chapter 11 in A Siva, J Kesselring, AJ Thompson (eds), Frontiers of Multiple Sclerosis, Vol. 2. London: Martin Dunitz.

Koopman W, Schweitzer A (1999) The journey to multiple sclerosis: a qualitative study, Journal of Neuroscience Nursing 31(1): 17–26.

Kraft GH (1986) Disability, disease duration and rehabilitation service needs in multiple sclerosis: patient perspectives, Archives of Physical Medicine and Rehabilitation 67: 164–78.

Krupp LB, Alverez LA, LaRocca NG, Scheinberg LC (1988) Fatigue in multiple sclerosis, Archives of Neurology 45: 435–7.

Krupp LB, Coyle PK, Doscher C, Miller A et al. (1995) Fatigue therapy in MS: results of a double-blind, randomised, parallel trial of amantadine, pemoline and placebo, Neurology 45: 1956–61.

Kurtzke JF (1983) Rating neurologic impairment in multiple sclerosis: an expanded disability status scale (EDSS), Neurology 33: 1444–52.

Kurtzke JF, Gudmundsson KR, Bergmann S (1982) Multiple sclerosis in Iceland: I. Evidence of a post war epidemic, Neurology 32: 143–50.

Kurtzke JF, Hyllested K (1988) Validity of the epidemics of multiple sclerosis in the Faro islands, Neuroepidemiology 7: 190–227.

Lance JW (1980) Symposium synopsis. In RG Feldman, RR Young, WP Koella (eds), Spasticity: Disordered Motor Control. Chicago: Year Book Medical Publishers, pp. 485–94.

Langdon DW (1997) Cognitive dysfunction in multiple sclerosis: what are we measuring and why does it matter? Chapter 19 in AJ Thompson, C Polman, R Hohlfeld (eds), Multiple Sclerosis: Clinical Challenges and Controversies. London: Martin Dunitz.

Lassmann H (1998) Pathology of multiple sclerosis. In A Compston, G Ebers, H Lassman, I McDonald et al. (eds), McAlpines Multiple Sclerosis, 3rd edn. London: Churchill Livingstone.

Lauer K (1997) Diet and multiple sclerosis, Neurology 49 (Suppl 2): S55–61.

Lechtenberg R (1995) The MS Fact Book. 2nd edn. Philadelphia: FA Davies.

Leviæ Z, Dujmoviæ I, Druloviæ J, Pekmezoiæ T et al. (1999) Prognosis in multiple sclerosis, Neurology, Psychiatry and Brain Research 6: 181–90.

Lilius HG, Valtonen EJ, Wikstrom J (1976) Sexual problems in patients suffering from multiple sclerosis, Scandinavian Journal of the Society of Medicine 4: 41–4.

Lublin FD, Reingold SC (1996) Defining the clinical course of multiple sclerosis: results of an international survey, Neurology 46: 907–11.

Lublin FD, Whitaker JN, Eidelman BH, Miller AE et al. (1996) Management of patients receiving interferon 1b for multiple sclerosis: report of a consensus conference, Neurology 46: 12–18.

McAlpine D, Compston N, Lumsden C (1955) Multiple Sclerosis. Edinburgh: Churchill Livingstone.

McCabe MP, McDonald E, Deeks AA, Vowels LM et al. (1996) The impact of multiple sclerosis on sexuality and relationships, Journal of Sexual Research 33(3): 241–8.

McDonald WI (1993) The dynamics of multiple sclerosis: the Charcot Lecture, Journal of Neurology 240: 28–36.

McDonald WI (1998) Diagnostic methods and investigations. In A Compston, G Ebers, H Lassman, I McDonald et al. (eds), McAlpines Multiple Sclerosis, 3rd edn. London: Churchill Livingstone.

McDonald WI, Thompson AJ (1997) How many kinds of multiple sclerosis are there? Chapter 3 in AJ Thompson, C Polman, R Hohlfeld (eds), Multiple Sclerosis: Clinical Challenges and Controversies. London: Martin Dunitz.

McDonald WI, Compston A, Ebers G, Goodkin D et al. (2001) Recommended diagnostic criteria for multiple sclerosis: guidelines from the international panel on the diagnosis of multiple sclerosis, Annals of Neurology 50: 121–7.

McDonnell GV, Hawkins SA (1996) Primary progressive multiple sclerosis: a distinct syndrome?, Multiple Sclerosis 2: 137–41.

McFarland G, McFarlane E (1997) Pain. In Nursing Diagnosis and Intervention, 3rd edn, Mosby, pp. 513–23.

McGuinness SD, Peters S (1999) The diagnosis of multiple sclerosis: Peplau's interpersonal relations model in practice, Rehabilitation Nursing 24(1): 30–3.

Mahoney F, Barthel DW (1965) Functional evaluation: The Barthel Index, Maryland State Medical Journal 14: 61–5.

Maloni HW (2000) Pain in multiple sclerosis: an overview of its nature and management, Journal of Neuroscience Nursing 32(3): 139–44.

Marie P (1884) Sclerose en plaques et maladies infecteuses, Progr. Med. Paris 12: 287–9.

Medaer R (1979) Does the history of multiple sclerosis go back as far as the 14th century?, Acta Neurol. Scandinavia 60: 189–92.

Medaer R, Stinissen P, Truyen L, Ravs J et al. (1995) Depletion of myelin basic protein autoreactive T cells by T cell vaccination: a pilot trial in multiple sclerosis, Lancet 346: 807–8.

Melia D (1998) Spasticity, Professional Nurse 13(12): 858–61.

Metz LM, McGuinness SD, Harris C (1998) Urinary tract infections may trigger relapse in multiple sclerosis, Axon 19(4): 67–70.

Minden SL (1992) Psychotherapy for people with multiple sclerosis, Journal of Neuropsychiatry 4: 198–213.

Mohr DC, Goodkin DE, Likosky W, Gatto N et al. (1997) Treatment of depression improves adherence to beta interferon 1b therapy for multiple sclerosis, Archives of Neurology 54: 531–3.

Moos RH, Shaefer JA (1984) The Crisis of Physical Illness: an Overview and Conceptual Approach.1. Coping with Physical Illness: 2. New Perspectives. New York: Plenum Press.

Morgante L (1997) Hope: a unifying concept for nursing care in multiple sclerosis. Chapter 14 in J Halper, N Holland (eds), Multiple Sclerosis: Comprehensive Nursing Care in Multiple Sclerosis. New York: Demos Vermande.

Moulin D, Foley K, Ebers G (1988) Pain syndromes in multiple sclerosis, Neurology 38: 1830–34.

MS Society (1997) Symptom Management Survey. MS Society of Great Britain and Northern Ireland and Athena Neurosciences.

Murray TJ (1995) The psychological aspect of multiple sclerosis, Neurologic Clinics 13(1): 197–223.

Mushlin AI, Mooney C, Grow V, Phelps CE (1994) The value of diagnostic information to patients with suspected multiple sclerosis, Archives of Neurology 51: 67–72.

Namey MA (1997) Management of elimination dysfunction. In J Halper, N Holland (eds), Comprehensive Nursing Care in Multiple Sclerosis. New York: Demos Vermande.

Nieves J, Cosman F, Herbert J, Shen V et al. (1994) High prevalence of vitamin D deficiency and reduced bone mass in multiple sclerosis, Neurology 44: 1687–92.

Norman JE, Kurtzke JF, Beebe GW (1983) Epidemiology of multiple sclerosis in US veterans: latitude, climate and risk of multiple sclerosis, Journal of Chronic Diseases 36: 551–9.

Noseworthy JH, Gold R, Hartung HP (1999) Treatment of multiple sclerosis: recent trials and future perspectives, Current Opinion in Neurology 279–93.

Orem D (1990) Concepts of Practice, 3rd edn. New York: McGraw Hill.

Owen DK, Lewith G, Stephens CR (2001) Can doctors respond to patients increasing interest in complementary and alternative medicine?, BMJ 322: 154–8.

Padma-Nathan H, Hellstrom W, Kaiser FE, Labasky RF et al. (1997) Treatment of men with erectile dysfunction with transurethral alprostadil, New England Journal of Medicine 336: 1–7.

Panitch H (1997) The importance of viral infections and vaccinations in multiple sclerosis. Chapter 9 in AJ Thompson, C Polman, R Hohlfeld (eds), Multiple Sclerosis: Clinical Challenges and Controversies. London: Martin Dunitz.

Panitch HS, Hirsch RL, Schindler J, Johnson KP (1987) Treatment of multiple sclerosis with gamma interferon: exacerbation's associated with activation of the immune system, Neurology 37: 1097–1102.

Panitch HS, Beuer CT (1993) Clinical trials of interferons in multiple sclerosis: what have we learned?, J. Neuroimmunology 46: 155–64.

Parkin D, McNamee P, Jacoby A, Miller P et al. (1998) A cost-utility analysis of beta interferon for multiple sclerosis, Health Technology A2(4).

Paty DW, Hartung HP (1999) Management of relapsing-remitting multiple sclerosis: diagnosis and treatment guidelines, European Journal of Neurology 6(S1): S6.

Petajan JH, Gappmaier E, White AT, Spencer MK et al. (1996) Impact of aerobic training on fitness and quality of life in multiple sclerosis, Annals of Neurology 39: 432–41.

Petkau J, White R (1997) Neutralising antibodies and the efficacy of beta interferon 1b in relapsing-remitting multiple sclerosis, Multiple Sclerosis 3: 402.

Pillemer K, Suitor JJ (1996) 'It takes one to help one': effects of similar others on the well being of caregivers, Journal of Gerontology 51b: s250–s257.

Pitzalis C, Sharrack B, Gray IA, Lee A et al. (1997) Comparison of the effects of oral versus intravenous methylprednisolone regimens on peripheral T lymphocyte adhesion molecule expression, T cell subsets, distribution and TNF alpha concentrations in multiple sclerosis, Journal of Neuroimmunology 74: 62–8.

Poser M (1995) Viking voyages: the origin of multiple sclerosis? an essay in medical history, Acta Neurol. Scandinavia Suppl 16(1): 11–22.

Poser CM, Paty DW, Scheinberg L, McDonald WI et al. (1983) New diagnostic criteria for multiple sclerosis: guidelines for research protocols, Annals of Neurology 13: 227–31.

Price GB (1997) Advocacy. Chapter 13 in J Halper, N Holland (eds), Comprehensive Nursing Care in Multiple Sclerosis. New York: Demos Vermande.

Prineas JW, Barnard RO, Kwon EE, Sharer LR et al. (1993) Multiple sclerosis: remyelination of nascent lesions, Annals of Neurology 33: 137–51.

PRISMS Study Group (1998) Randomised double blind, placebo-controlled study of interferon beta 1a in relapsing-remitting multiple sclerosis, Lancet 352: 1498–1504.

R&D Focus (1994) Drug News, 13 June, p. 10, IMS World Publications.

Rabins PV, Brooks BR, O'Donnell P, Pearlson GD et al. (1986) Structural brain correlates of emotional disorder in multiple sclerosis, Brain 109: 585–97.

Rammohan KW, Rosenberg JH, Pollak CP, Lynn DJ et al. (2000) Provigil shows promise as a treatment for fatigue in MS. MS Update. From Science to Patient Care 2(1): 7–8.

Rao SM, Leo GJ, Bernadin L, Unverzagt F (1991) Cognitive dysfunction in multiple sclerosis 1. Frequency, patterns and predictions, Neurology 41: 685–91.

Rapp NS, Gilroy J, Lerner AM (1995) Role of bacterial infection in exacerbation of multiple sclerosis, American Journal of Physical Medicine and Rehabilitation 74: 415–18.

RCN (2000) Sexuality and Sexual Health in Nursing Practice.

Remick RA, Sadovnick AD (1997) Depression and suicide in multiple sclerosis. Chapter 18 in AJ Thompson, C Polman, R Hohlfeld (eds), Multiple Sclerosis: Clinical Challenges and Controversies. London: Martin Dunitz.

Revesz T, Kidd D, Thompson AJ, Barnard RO et al. (1994) A comparison of the pathology of primary and secondary multiple sclerosis, Brain 117(4): 759–65.

Riise T (1997) Is the incidence of multiple sclerosis increasing? In AJ Thompson, C Polman, R Hohlfeld (eds), Multiple Sclerosis: Clinical Challenges and Controversies. London: Martin Dunitz.

Ritvo PG, Fisk JD, Archibald CJ et al. (1992) A model of mental health in patients with multiple sclerosis, Canadian Psychology 33: 391.

Robertson NP, Fraser M, Deans J, Clayton D et al. (1996) Age adjusted recurrence risks for relatives of patients with multiple sclerosis, Brain 119: 449–55.

Robertson WF (1899) On a new method of obtaining a black reaction in certain tissue elements of the central nervous system (platinum method), Scottish Medical and Surgical Journal 4: 23–30.

Robinson I (1991) The context and consequences of communicating the diagnosis of multiple sclerosis: some brief findings from a survey of 900 patients, Current Concepts in Multiple Sclerosis, Proceedings of the 6th Congress of the European Committee for Treatment and Research in Multiple Sclerosis (ECTRIMS) Tubingen 11–13 October, pp. 17–22.

Ron MA, Logsdail SJ (1989) Psychiatric morbidity in multiple sclerosis: a clinical and MRI study, Psychological Medicine 19: 887–95.

Roper N, Logan W, Tierney A (1996) The Elements of Nursing, 4th edn. Edinburgh: Churchill Livingstone.

Rothwell PM, McDowell Z, Wong CK, Dorman PJ (1997) Doctors and patients don't agree: cross sectional study of patients and doctors perceptions and assessments of disability in multiple sclerosis, BMJ 314: 1580–3.

Rudge P (1999) The value of natural history studies of multiple sclerosis, Brain 122(4): 591–2.

Runmarker B, Anderson O (1993) Prognostic factors in a multiple sclerosis incidence cohort with 25 years of follow up, Brain 116(1): 117–34.

Runmarker B, Anderson O (1995) Pregnancy is associated with a lower risk of onset and a better prognosis in multiple sclerosis, Brain 118: 253–61.

Sadovnick AD, Ebers GC (1993) Epidemiology of multiple sclerosis: a critical overview, Canadian Journal of Neurological Science 20: 17–29.

Sadovnick AD, Baird PA, Ware RH (1988) Multiple sclerosis: updated risks for relatives, American Journal of Medical Genetics 29: 533–41.

Sadovnick AD, Eisen GC, Wilson RW, Paty DW (1991) Life expectancy in patients attending multiple sclerosis clinics, Neurology 41: 1193–96.

Sadovnick AD, Armstrong H, Rice GPA, Bulman D et al. (1993) A population based study of multiple sclerosis in twins: update, Annals of Neurology 33: 281–5.

Sadovnick AD, Remick RA, Allen J, Swartz E et al. (1996) Depression and multiple sclerosis, Neurology 46: 628–32.

Schapiro RT, Schneider DM (1997) Symptom management. Chapter 3 in J Halper, NJ Holland (eds), Comprehensive Nursing Care in Multiple Sclerosis. New York: Demos Vermande.

Schapiro RT, Baumhefner RW, Tourtellotte WW (1997) Multiple sclerosis: a clinical viewpoint to management. Chapter 23 in CS Raine, HF McFarland, WW Tourtellotte (eds), Multiple Sclerosis Clinical and Pathogenetic Basis. London: Chapman & Hall.

Schiffer RB, Wineman NM (1990) Antidepressant pharmacotherapy of depression associated with multiple sclerosis, American Journal of Psychiatry 147: 1493–7.

Schiffer RB, Hendon RM, Rudick RA (1985) Treatment of pathological laughing and weeping with amitriptyline, New England Journal of Medicine 412: 1480.

Schild HH (1990) MRI Made Easy. Berlin: H Heenemann GmbH & Co.

Schwid SR, Goodman AD, Puzas EJ, McDermott MP et al. (1996) Sporadic corticosteroid pulses and osteoporosis in multiple sclerosis, Archives of Neurology 53: 753–7.

Scolding N (1999) Long term repair in MS, Phil Trans R. Soc. London B 354: 1711–20.

Scott G (2000) NICE agrees to reconsider beta-interferon proposals, Nursing Standard 15(9): 8.

Sellebjerg F, Frederikson JL, Nielsen PM, Olesen J (1998) Double-blind, randomised, placebo controlled study of oral high dose methyl prednisolone in attacks of MS, Neurology 51: 529–34.

Sharrack B, Hughes RAC (1999) The Guy's Neurological Disability Scale (GNDS): a new disability measure for multiple sclerosis, Multiple Sclerosis 5(4): 223–33.

Sheean G (1998a) A pathophysiology of spasticity. Chapter 3 in G Sheean (ed.), Spasticity Rehabilitation. Churchill Communications, Europe.

Sheean G (1998b) The treatment of spasticity with botulinum toxin. Chapter 9 in G Sheean (ed.), Spasticity Rehabilitation. Churchill Communications, Europe.

Siev-Ner I, Gamus D, Lerner-Gevea L et al. (1997) Reflexology treatment relieves symptoms of multiple sclerosis: a randomised controlled study, Focus on Alternative and Complementary Therapy 2(4): 196.

Sinclair A, Dickinson E (1998) Effective Practice in Rehabilitation: The Evidence of Systematic Reviews. London: Kings Fund.

Sipe JC, Knobler RL, Braheny SL, Rice GP et al. (1984) A neurologic rating scale (NRS) for use in multiple sclerosis, Neurology 34: 1368–72.

Smythe MD, Peacock WJ (2000) The surgical treatment of spasticity, Muscle and Nerve, Feb.: 153–63.

Snow BJ, Tsui JK C, Bhatt MH, Varelas M et al. (1990) Treatment of spasticity with botulinum toxin: a double blind study, Annals of Neurology 28: 512–15.

Sørensen PS, Wanscher B, Jensen CV, Schreiber K et al. (1998) Intravenous immunoglobulin G reduces MRI activity in relapsing-remitting MS, Neurology 50: 1273–81.

SPECTRIMS Study Group (2000) Secondary progressive efficacy clinical trial of Rebif in MS. Presented at the American Academy of Neurology 52nd Annual meeting. San Diego, USA, 29 April–6 May.

Stevenson VL, Miller DH, Leary SM, Rovaris M et al. (2000) One year follow up study of primary and transitional progressive multiple sclerosis, Journal of Neurology, Neurosurgery and Psychiatry 68: 713–18.

Targett MP, Sussman J, Scolding N, O'Leary MT et al. (1996) Failure to achieve remyelination of demyelinated rat axons following transplantation of glial cells obtained from the adult human brain, Neuropathology and Applied Neurobiology 22: 199–206.

Thompson AJ (1998) Spasticity rehabilitation. Chapter 5 in G Sheean (ed.), Spasticity Rehabilitation. Churchill Communications, Europe.

Thompson AJ, Hobart JC (1998) Multiple sclerosis: assessment of disability and disability scales, Journal of Neurology 245: 189–96.

Thompson AJ, Polman CH, Miller DH, McDonald WI et al. (1997) Primary progressive multiple sclerosis, Brain 120(6): 1085–96.

Thompson AJ, Montalban X, Barkhof F, Brochet B et al. (2000) Diagnostic criteria for primary progressive multiple sclerosis: a position paper, Annals of Neurology 47: 831–5.

Thorogood M, Hannaford PC (1998) The influence of oral contraceptives on the risk of multiple sclerosis, British Journal of Obstetrics and Gynaecology 195: 1296–9.

Trapp BD, Ransohoff RM, Fisher E, Rudick RA (1999) Neurodegeneration in multiple sclerosis: relationship to neurological disability, Neuroscientist 5: 48–57.

Tremlett HL, Luscombe DK, Wiles CM (1998) Use of corticosteroids in multiple sclerosis by consultant neurologists in the United Kingdom, Journal of Neurology, Neurosurgery and Psychiatry 65: 362–5.

Tremlett HL, Wiles CM (1999) Oral or intravenous: the evidence for corticosteroids in MS relapse, Progress in Neurology and Psychiatry 3(1): 19–23.

Trevelyan J (1993) Acupuncture, Nursing Times 89(28): 26–8.

UKCC (1997) PREP and You. London: UKCC.

UK Tizanidine Trial Group (1994) A double blind, placebo controlled trial of tizanidine in the treatment of spasticity caused by multiple sclerosis, Neurology 44(Suppl 9): S70–S78.

US Modafinil in Narcolepsy Multicentre Study Group (2000) Randomised trial of modafinil as a treatment for the excessive daytime somnolence of narcolepsy, Neurology 54: 1166–75.

Üstün TB, Leonardi M (1998) The revision of the international classification of impairments, disabilities and handicaps (ICIDH-2), European Journal of Neurology 5(S2): S31–S32.

Valleroy MR, Kraft GH (1984) Sexual dysfunction in multiple sclerosis, Archives of Physical Medical Rehabilitation 65: 125–8.

van Overstaten AR (1999) The patients role in the improvement of care, Multiple Sclerosis 5(4): 302–5.

Vleugels L, Pfennings L, Pouwer F, Cohen L et al. (1998) Psychological functioning in primary progressive versus secondary progressive multiple sclerosis, British Journal Medical Psychology 71(1): 99–106.

Wade DT (1996) Epidemiology of disabling neurological disease: how and why does disability occur?, Journal of Neurology, Neurosurgery and Psychiatry 61: 242–9.

Walker PW, Cole JO, Gardner EA, Hughes AR et al. (1993) Improvement in Fluoxetine associated sexual dysfunction in patients switched to buproprion, Journal of Clinical Psychiatry 54: 459–65.

Walsh M (1998) Models and critical pathways in clinical nursing. Conceptual Frameworks for Care Planning, 2nd edn. London: Ballière Tindall.

Walsh M, Ford P (1989) Nursing Rituals, Research and Rational Actions. Oxford: Butterworth-Heinemann.

Webb RJ, Lawson AL, Neal DE (1990) Clean intermittent self-catheterisation in 172 adults, British Journal of Urology 65: 20–3.

Weinshenker BG (1997) The natural history of multiple sclerosis. Chapter 6 in CS Raine, HF McFarland, WW Tourtellotte (eds), Multiple Sclerosis Clinical and Pathogenetic Basis. London: Chapman & Hall.

Weinshenker BG et al. (1998) The natural history of multiple sclerosis: Update 1998, Seminars in Neurology 18(3): 301–7.

Weinshenker BG, Penman M, Bass B, Ebers GC et al. (1992) A double blind, randomised, crossover trial of pemoline in fatigue associated with multiple sclerosis, Neurology 42: 1468–71.

Wells A (1997) Cognitive Therapy of Anxiety Disorders. London: Wiley.

Werring DJ, Thompson AJ (1998) Medical & surgical treatment of spasticity. Chapter 8 in G Sheean (ed.), Spasticity Rehabilitation. Churchill Communications, Europe.

Westbrook MT, Viney LL (1982) Psychological reactions to the onset of chronic illness, Social Science Medicine 16: 899–905.

Weston A (1993) Challenging assumptions, Nursing Times 89(18): 26–31.

Wiles CM, Newcombe RG, Fuller KJ, Shaw S et al. (2001) Controlled randomised crossover trial of the effects of physiotherapy on mobility in chronic multiple sclerosis, Journal of Neurology, Neurosurgery and Psychiatry 70: 174–9.

Wilkinson K (1996) The concept of hope in life-threatening illness, Professional Nurse 11(10): 659–61.

Wilson M, Coates D (1996) Infection control and urine drainage bag design, Professional Nurse 11(4): 245–52.

Witherington R (1989) Vacuum constriction device for management of erectile impotence, Journal of Urology 141: 320–2.

Wolinsky J (2000) Glatiramer acetate. Chapter 5 in CP Hawkins C, JS Wolinsky (eds) Principles of Treatments in Multiple Sclerosis. Oxford: Butterworth-Heinemann.

Young C (2000) Symptomatic management: ataxia, tremor and fatigue. Chapter 14 in CP Hawkins, JS Wolinsky (eds), Principles of Treatments in Multiple Sclerosis. Oxford: Butterworth-Heinemann.

Young IR, Hall AS, Pallis CA, Legg NJ et al. (1981) Nuclear magnetic resonance imaging of the brain in multiple sclerosis, Lancet II: 1063–6.

Zhang JW, Medaer R, Stinissen P, Hafler D et al. (1993) MHC restricted clonotypic depletion of human myelin basic protein – reactive T cells by T cell vaccination, Science 261: 1451–4.

Index

acupuncture 180
advocacy 157–158
age of onset 11
alcohol 104, 110,122
amantadine 81
amitriptyline 93,109,122
anatomy
    of the blood brain barrier 14,16–18
    of the bowel 116–117
    of the central nervous system 14–16,
       72–75
    of the cranial nerves 23–24, 75
    of the urinary system 101–102, 128,
       129
anxiety 175–177
aromatherapy 180
assessment 151–156
    of bladder function 105–107
    of fatigue 77–79
    of sexual function 122–123, 127–128
astrocytes 14,16
ataxia 25, 73, 83, 96
attention, impaired 148–149
auditory evoked potentials 31
Avonex *see* interferons

Babinski reflex 26
Baclofen *see* lioresal
balance 24, 26, 73, 83
banding 89, 90
Benefits 167–168
Benign MS 46–47
Betaferon *see* interferons
bladder symptoms
    assessment of 105–107
    exacerbating factors 104–105

frequency 102, 108–109
hesitancy 103
incomplete emptying 103
incontinence 103, 108–109, 199
nocturia 102, 109
self help 110
treatment of 107–109
urgency 102–103, 108–109
urinary tract infection 103, 107–108,
    114, 169
body image 97, 105, 129
Botulinum toxin 189–190
bowel function 116–120, 128
bowel symptoms 117–120
    constipation 117–119
    incontinence 119–120
    self-help 118
    treatment 118
Brain, Russell 4

cannabis 94, 122, 188, 208
carbamazepine 93, 122
carers 130, 184, 187, 200–201, 203–204
Carers' Association 201
Carswell, Robert 1,2
catheters 114–116, 129
    blockage of 115–116
    intermittent self-catheterisation 108,
      112–114
    long-term 114
    supra-pubic 116
causative agents (potential)
    chance 11
    diet 13
    environmental 13, 14
    infective 2, 8,11,13

cerebral atrophy 46
Charcot, Jean-Martin 3, 4, 137
children with MS 11
clinical guidelines 205
cognitive impairment 129, 137–138,
　　145–149
　problem solving 147
cold feet 97
complimentary therapies 177–183
conduction block 5,18
Continence Advisor 111, 114
contraception 133
constipation 117–119
co-ordination 26
counselling 40, 142
Copaxone *see* glatiramer acetate
coping skills 33–34, 42, 43–44, 92, 148,
　　161, 163–164, 173–177
Cruveillhier 2

dantrolene 87
D'Este, Augustus 3
demyelination 18
depression 121, 138–142
　treatment of 141–142
desmopressin 109
detrusia dysfunction 103–104
detrusitol 109, 128
diagnosis
　communicating a diagnosis 33–35
　criteria for diagnosis 31–33
　following pregnancy 136
　impact on patient 35–38
　interdisciplinary team and 38–40
　neurological examination 22–26
　patient history 22
　peak age of 1
　primary care 20–21
　psychological impact of 35–38
　referral for 21
diazepam 87
diet 13, 171–172, 199
　vitamin D3 13
Dietician 111, 172
disability 50–54
　medical and social models of 51
　WHO Key Terms 50
Disability Discrimination Act 164–166
diuretics 97
double vision 95

driving 168
dysarthria 23, 24, 96
dysasthesia 89–90, 122, 127, 129, 199
dysphagia 96, 196–198
dysphasia 23

EDSS 52–53, 56–57
employment 164–166
end-stage MS 201–204
epidemiology of MS 7–14
　confounding factors 8–9
　frequency of MS 9
　incidence of MS 4, 9
　male to female ratio 11
　prevalence of MS 9, 10, 14 21
erectile dysfunction 121–127
euphoria 144–145
evidence based practice 162
evoked potentials 31
exercise 92, 172–173

faecal incontinence 119– 120, 199
fatigue 76–82, 109, 122, 128
　assessment of 77–79
　depression and 138
　patients role 80
　pathophysiology of 77
FIM/FAM 53
foot drop 25, 85–86

Gabapentin *see* neurontin
general practitioner 20–21, 38, 178
genetic factors 11, 13, 134
　migration studies 12–13
　twin studies 12
geographical distribution 9–10
　population migrations 10, 12
　Vikings, influence on 10
glatiramer acetate 56–58, 64, 135
　side-effects 64–65
　trial design 57–58
gliosis 18
grieving 37, 137, 138
Guy's Neurological Disability Scale 54

headache 89
heat 80,170 *see also* temperature control
Henderson, Virginia 150
herbalism 179
homeopathy 179

hesitancy 103
hope 158–160
hyperbaric oxygen 181

IgG Index 30–31, 32
Imipramine 93,109
Immunoglobulin G, intravenous 70
immunology 14, 16–17
    cytokines 17, 18
    imunoglobulins 16, 30
    T cells 16–17
incidence of MS 4, 9
incontinence, bladder 103, 108–109
incontinence, bowel 119–120
interferons 6–7, 17, 52–53, 55–70, 135,
    205
    commencing treatment 60–62
    impact on patients 59
    management of side effects 62–69
        depression 65–66
        injection site reactions 64–65
        trouble shooting 66–69
    neutralising antibodies 69–70
    NICE 59–60, 158
    pregnancy 61
    prescribing of 58–60
    QALY 58
    secondary progressive MS 58
    stopping treatment 69
    trial design 56–58
intermittent self-catheterisation 108,
    112–114

laxatives 118
libido, reduced 127
Lidwina, Saint 1–2
life expectancy 201–202
life long learning 159–160
lioresal 86–87, 191–193
lumbar puncture 28–31
    care of patient undergoing 29
    results of 30

McAlpine, Douglas 5
magnetic resonance imaging (MRI) 6, 27,
    28, 32
    care of patient undergoing 27–28
    Gadolinium DTPA 27
Marburg's MS 47
massage 92, 180

memory 145–147
microglia 15
mitoxantrone 71
mobility 82–87
modafanil 208
models of nursing 153–156
mood swings 142–145
MS Research trust 40
MS Society 5, 8, 35, 39, 40, 175, 205
    'Standards of healthcare' 7, 22, 34, 40,
        205
MS specialist nurse 6, 21, 35, 39, 60–62
MUSE 124–125
myelin 3, 14, 15, 18
    nodes of ranvier 15

NARCOMS 49
neuroglia 4, 18
neurologist 33–35, 39, 86–87, 92–94
neurones 14–15
neurontin 93
nocturia 102, 109
numbness *see* dysasthesia
nurse 77–80, 84, 91, 92, 109–110,
    130–134, 139–141, 150–162
nystagmus 24, 96

occupational therapist 39, 80, 86, 94, 111,
    147, 188
oligoclonal bands 31, 32
oligodendrocytes 4, 14, 18
optic neuritis 24, 89, 95
Orkneys 10–11
orthotist 85
oxybutinin 109, 128

pain 87–95, 122
    assessment of 91–92
    coping strategies 92
    musculoskeletal 90
palliative care 184
percutaneous endoscopic gastrostomy
    (PEG) 197–198
Peplau's interpersonal relations model
    155
pemoline 82
physiotherapist 39, 81, 84, 94, 111, 173,
    186, 188, 208, 209
phenol block 190–191
plaques 17, 18, 28, 73

P-LI- SS-IT model 131–132
Poser criteria 32
post mortem studies 41
pregnancy 132–136
    medication and, 134–135
prevalence 9, 10, 14, 21
primary progressive MS 33, 44–46
    diagnosing 45
    differences from secondary progressive
        MS 45–46
prognosis 7, 42, 48–50
progressive relapsing MS 45
proprioception 25
psychologist 95

rating scales 50–54
    EDSS 52, 53
    Guy's neurological disability scale 54
    patients perspective 53, 54
    Scripp's neurological rating scale
Rebif *see* interferons
reflexology 180
rehabilitation 156–157, 208–209
relapse 32, 42
    management of 98
    trigger factors 169–171
relapsing remitting MS 43
relationships 130
relaxation techniques 92, 181, 182
remission 19
remyelination 4, 5, 18, 206–207
Rindfleisch 4
risk of developing MS 11, 12, 14
role change 130
Romberg's test 26

Scripp's neurological rating scale 53
secondary progressive MS 17, 44, 58
sexual function
    assessment of 122–123, 127–128
    erectile dysfunction 123–127
    priapism 126
    treatment of 123–128
    women and, 128–130

sildenafil 123–124, 128
skin care 120, 186, 198–200
smoking 104, 110, 122
social worker 25, 39
speech *see* dysarthria
speech and language therapist 96
spasms 84, 90, 122
spasticity 121, 184–194
    aggravating factors 186, 187–188
    impact on individual 186
    management of 187–194
    surgical intervention 193–194
stem cells 208–209
steroids 98–100
    management of side-effects 100
stress 20, 170–171
suicide 141, 202
swallowing *see* dysphagia
swollen ankles 97–98

T'ai Chi 181
teaching 158–160
team working 156–157
temperature control 96, 97
Tegretol *see* carbamazepine
tizanadine 87
transition phase 43
tremor 73, 194–196
trigeminal neuralgia 24, 89, 93

vaccinations 169–170, 207
vacuum devices 126–127
Viagra *see* sildenafil
visual disturbances 93–96
visual evoked potentials 31, 33
vitamin B12 81
walking aids 85
weakness 83
Wellness model 163–164

Yoga 181
Yohimbine 128

Zanaflex *see* tizanadine